Copy Editor and Interior Design: Constance Santego
Book Layout: ©2017 BookDesignTemplates.com

Ordering Information:
Quantity sales. Special discounts are available on quantity purchases by corporations, associations, and others. For details, contact the "Special Sales Department" at the address above.

Trade paperback ISBN: 978-1-990062-20-9

eBook ISBN 978-1-990062-21-6

Created and published In Canada. Printed and bound in the United States of America

Published by Maximillian Enterprises
Kelowna, BC
Canada
www.constancesantego.ca

Scaling Beyond 6 Figures:

Strategies for Health & Wellness Professionals

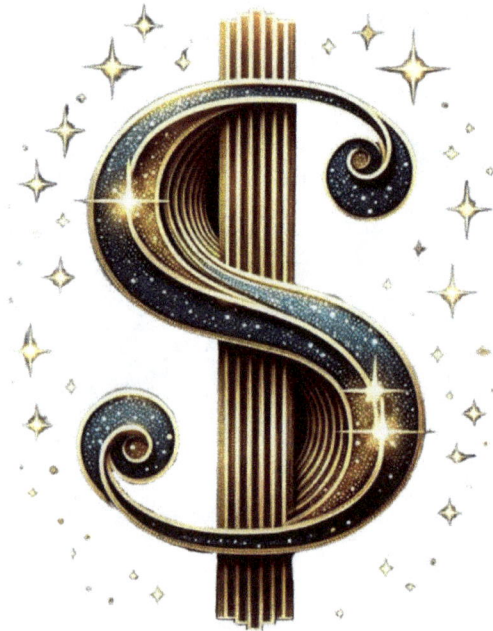

Dr. Constance Santego IV

Also, By Dr. Constance Santego

FICTION

THE NINE SPIRITUAL GIFTS SERIES:

Journey of a Soul – (Vol. 1 Michael)

Language of a Soul – (Vol. 2 Gabriel)

Prophecy of a Soul – (Vol. 3 Bath Kol)

Healing of a Soul – (Vol. 4 Raphael)

Miracles of a Soul – (Vol. 5 Hamied)

NON-FICTION

The Intuitive Life, The Gift of Prophecy, Third Edition

Your Persona... The Mask You Wear

Angelic Lifestyle, A Vibrant Lifestyle

Angelic Lifestyle 42-Day Energy Cleanse

Archangel Michael's Soul Retrieval Guide

Tesla and the Future of Energy Medicine

Bend, Don't Break: Finding Your Way Back To Abundance

SECRETS OF A HEALER, SERIES:

Magic of Aromatherapy (Vol. I)

Magic of Reflexology (Vol. II)

Magic of The Gifts (Vol. III)

Magic of Muscle Testing (Vol. IV)

Magic of Iridology (Vol. V)

Magic of Massage (Vol. VI)

Magic of Hypnotherapy (Vol. VII)

Magic of Reiki (Vol. VIII)

Magic of Advanced Aromatherapy (Vol. IX)

Magic of Esthetics (Vol. X)

FOR CHILDREN

I am Big Tonight. I Don't Need the Light!

SCALING BEYOND 6 FIGURES:

Strategies for Health & Wellness Professionals

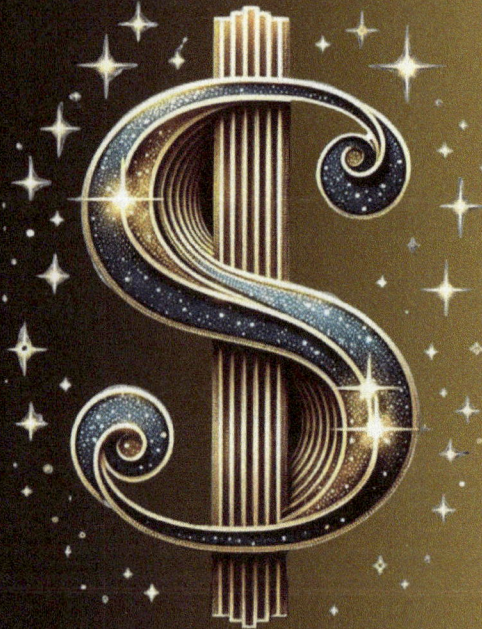

DR. CONSTANCE SANTEGO

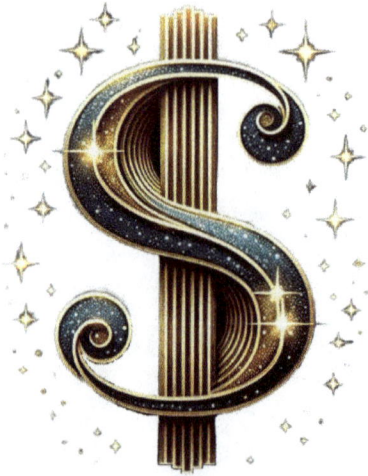

Dedication

I would like to dedicate this book to the space between, *which makes reality!*

Dr. Constance Santego x

Preface

Welcome to "Scaling Beyond 6 Figures: Strategies for Health & Wellness Professionals," a guide designed for the passionate healer, the visionary entrepreneur, and every holistic practitioner in between who dreams of making a profound impact while achieving financial prosperity. This book is born out of a recognition of the unique challenges and incredible opportunities that lie at the intersection of holistic health and business growth. It is an invitation to embark on a journey of transformation, not only for your practice but for the lives you touch.

In the realm of health and wellness, practitioners are often driven by a deep-seated desire to heal and help. Yet, the path to translating this noble intent into a sustainable, thriving business is seldom straightforward. The leap from being a practitioner to becoming a holistic entrepreneur entails a blend of passion, purpose, and practicality that this book aims to nurture and guide.

"Scaling Beyond 6 Figures" is more than a manua, it's a companion on your journey toward expanding your practice with integrity, innovation, and intent. It draws on the wisdom of seasoned professionals, the latest trends in holistic health and wellness, and actionable strategies for business development. Each chapter is crafted to address the core aspects of scaling a holistic health business—from building a solid foundation and embracing digital innovation to mastering the art of the pitch and securing investment with a purpose.

The heart of this book lies in its commitment to the principle that growth should never compromise the essence of holistic practice. Instead, it argues that scaling is an opportunity to amplify your impact, reach more individuals in need of healing, and contribute to the global shift toward a more holistic understanding of health and well-being.

As we navigate the pages together, you'll find case studies that inspire, strategies that empower, and insights that illuminate the path ahead. Whether you're an experienced practitioner looking to broaden your reach or a budding entrepreneur at the beginning of your holistic journey, this book offers the tools and inspiration needed to scale your business beyond six figures—mindfully, purposefully, and successfully.

I invite you to join me on this journey, to embrace the challenges and opportunities of holistic entrepreneurship, and to envision a future where your practice not only thrives financially but continues to make a profound difference in the world of health and wellness. Let's begin the journey to scale beyond six figures, together.

With warmth and encouragement,

Dr. Constance Santego

Contents

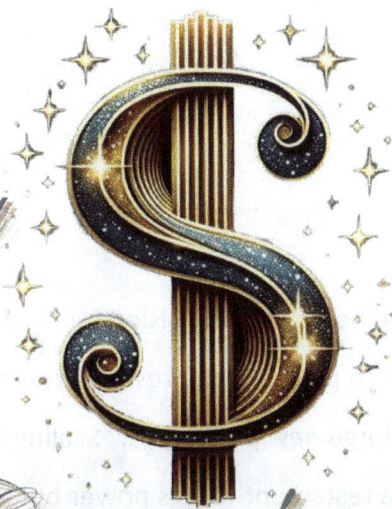

Your
Impact
is your
True Currency!

Introduction

The Power of Intent in Holistic Entrepreneurship:

In the heart of every visionary lies the power of intent—a force so potent it can reshape realities, elevate perceptions, and forge new paradigms. "Scaling Beyond 6 Figures" is not just a testament to this power but a strategic guide designed to unlock it, especially for those in the realm of holistic and alternative medicine. This book is a clarion call to wellness entrepreneurs ready to amplify their impact, credibility, and financial success to unparalleled heights.

Crafted with precision and passion by Dr. Constance Santego, this transformative work invites you on a journey where the essence of holistic well-being and the mechanics of business growth converge in perfect harmony. It challenges you to not only envision scaling your enterprise but to do so with a fervent intent that elevates the entire field of holistic and alternative medicine to newfound levels of respect and recognition.

At its core, "Scaling Beyond 6 Figures" dares to imagine a world where holistic practitioners stand shoulder to shoulder with the most celebrated entrepreneurs of our time—where being a millionaire or even a billionaire in the wellness industry is not an anomaly but a testament to the sector's value and impact. It's about recognizing the incredible potential within the wellness community to transform lives on a massive scale, backed by the same credibility and financial success attributed to traditional business moguls.

This book serves as your compass and companion on a journey to redefine success. Through insightful strategies, personal empowerment, and a deep dive into the art of intent, we will explore how to scale your business while honoring the principles that define holistic practice. You'll discover how to harness the power of intent to not only achieve financial milestones but also to shift societal perceptions, granting holistic and alternative medicine the credibility and esteem it richly deserves.

Prepare to challenge the status quo, to dream bigger, and to ignite a global shift in how holistic wellness is perceived and valued. "Scaling Beyond 6 Figures" is more than a roadmap to financial success; it's a blueprint for elevating the entire wellness industry, showcasing the profound power of intent and the boundless potential of those who wield it with conviction and clarity.

As we embark on this transformative journey, remember: the power to elevate holistic and alternative medicine, to achieve parity with the business elite, and to create a legacy of health, wealth, and well-being, begins with your intent. Let this book be the spark that ignites your path to unparalleled success.

Are you ready to witness the power of intent in action? To scale your practice beyond boundaries and elevate the field to unprecedented heights? Let's begin.

PART-1

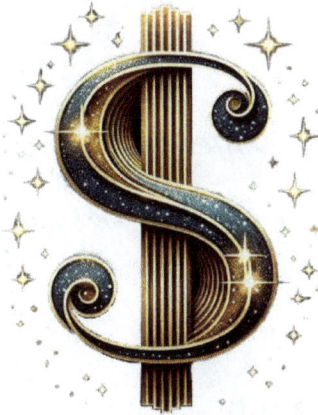

Cultivating a

Visionary

Mindset

Chapter 1

The Essence of Intent: Understanding and Harnessing Intent for Transformative Success

The Power of Intent

At the heart of every significant change and achievement lies intent. Intent is not merely about wanting something; it's the clarity and commitment behind your desires. It's the driving force that shapes your thoughts, guides your actions, and ultimately, manifests your reality. In the realm of holistic entrepreneurship, understanding and harnessing the power of intent can lead to transformative success—not just for you, but for the world around you.

Defining Intent

Intent goes beyond simple goal-setting. It encompasses the why behind what you do, imbuing your actions with purpose and direction. It's your inner compass, aligning your entrepreneurial journey with your core values and the impact you wish to create. When your business activities are powered by genuine intent, they resonate more deeply with others, attracting clients, partners, and opportunities that align with your vision.

Cultivating a Visionary Mindset

To harness intent, you must first cultivate a visionary mindset. This involves:

- Self-reflection: Understand your motivations, values, and the change you want to see through your business.
- Visualization: Regularly envision your success and the positive impact of your work. Visualization not only clarifies your intent but also prepares your subconscious to recognize and seize opportunities.
- Affirmation: Reinforce your intent with positive affirmations. Words have power; speaking your intent

out loud strengthens your belief in your ability to achieve it.

The Role of Mindfulness in Intent

Mindfulness is a critical tool for honing intent. By being present and fully engaged in the moment, you can better understand the needs of your clients, the shifts in the wellness industry, and the nuances of your business operations. Mindfulness helps maintain a clear focus on your intent, ensuring that your actions are deliberate and aligned with your goals.

Intent in Action

Putting intent into action involves several steps:

- Strategic Planning: Use your intent to guide your business strategy. Let it inform your decisions, from the services you offer to the way you market them.
- Consistent Application: Let intent drive your daily activities. Whether it's how you interact with clients or how you manage your team, every action should reflect your core intent.

- Adaptability: Be prepared to adjust your strategies as needed while staying true to your intent. The path to success is rarely linear, but a strong intent will keep you moving in the right direction.

The essence of intent is the recognition that your innermost desires and goals have the power to shape your entrepreneurial journey and the impact you make. By understanding and harnessing intent, you can transform your business into a vehicle for not only financial success but also for meaningful change in the holistic wellness community. This chapter sets the stage for cultivating a visionary mindset, a prerequisite for scaling your business beyond six figures while staying true to the principles of holistic well-being.

Self-reflection: Understanding Your Motivations, Values, and Desired Change

Step 1: Identify Your Core Values

Values are the guiding principles or fundamental beliefs that dictate behavior and action. They help determine what is important to an individual or organization, influencing decisions, actions, and priorities. Values serve as a compass that directs how a person or group interacts with others, approaches challenges, and makes choices, reflecting what is prioritized and cherished in life or business.

- List Your Values: **Start by listing values that resonate with you deeply. These could include integrity, compassion, innovation, sustainability, or wellness. Don't rush this process; take your time to truly connect with what matters most to you.**
- Prioritize: **Once you have a list, prioritize these values based on their significance to you. Which ones are absolutely non-negotiable in how you conduct your business and life?**

HOLISTIC AND ALTERNATIVE PRACTITIONERS often prioritize values that reflect their commitment to healing, wellness, and the interconnectedness of body, mind, and spirit. Typical values for someone in this field might include:

- o Compassion: Emphasizing empathy and a deep understanding of clients' experiences and needs.
- o Integrity: Adhering to ethical practices, honesty, and transparency in all interactions and treatments.
- o Holism: Recognizing the interdependence of all aspects of health—physical, mental, emotional, and spiritual—and treating the whole person rather than just symptoms.
- o Sustainability: Valuing and implementing practices that are sustainable for the planet and promote long-term wellness for individuals and communities.
- o Empowerment: Encouraging clients to take charge of their health and wellness, providing

them with the knowledge and tools to make informed decisions.

o   Inclusivity: Welcoming and respecting clients from all backgrounds and walks of life, understanding that everyone's path to wellness is unique.

o   Continuous Learning: Committing to ongoing education and exploration of new and traditional healing modalities to provide the best care possible.

o   Mindfulness: Practicing and promoting mindfulness and presence as essential components of health and healing.

o   Connection: Building strong, supportive relationships with clients, other practitioners, and the community, recognizing the power of connection in the healing process.

o   Innovation: Being open to exploring and integrating innovative approaches and technologies that enhance holistic healing practices.

These values not only guide their practices and interactions with clients but also shape the business models and community engagements of holistic and alternative practitioners.

SUCCESSFUL BUSINESSPEOPLE, including millionaires and entrepreneurs, often share a core set of values that drive their success. These values not only influence their decision-making and leadership styles but also define their approach to business and personal growth:

- o Integrity: Committing to honesty, ethical practices, and transparency in all business dealings.
- o Resilience: Demonstrating the ability to bounce back from failures, setbacks, and challenges, viewing them as opportunities for learning and growth.
- o Innovation: Constantly seeking new ideas, approaches, and solutions to stay ahead in a competitive market.
- o Determination: Possessing a strong will to achieve goals, regardless of obstacles, and persisting in the face of adversity.

- o Discipline: **Applying self-control and consistency to work habits, financial decisions, and time management.**
- o Vision: **Having a clear, compelling vision for the future of the business and the ability to communicate this vision to inspire others.**
- o Adaptability: **Being flexible and open to change, adjusting strategies in response to market shifts and new opportunities.**
- o Leadership: **Inspiring and motivating teams, fostering a positive and productive work environment, and leading by example.**
- o Customer Focus: **Prioritizing customer satisfaction and value creation, understanding that customers are the foundation of any successful business.**
- o Continuous Learning: **Embracing lifelong learning, seeking out mentorship, and remaining open to feedback for personal and professional development.**
- o Networking: **Building and nurturing relationships with peers, mentors, and industry leaders to open doors to new opportunities and collaborations.**
- o Philanthropy: **Giving back to the community and engaging in social responsibility initiatives,**

understanding the importance of making a positive impact beyond business success.

These values contribute to the creation of a strong, sustainable business and a legacy of success that goes beyond financial achievements.

BRIDGING THE VALUES OF HOLISTIC PRACTITIONERS WITH THOSE OF SUCCESSFUL BUSINESSPEOPLE creates a powerful synergy that can lead to unparalleled success, both personally and professionally. Here's how these seemingly distinct sets of values can connect and complement each other in the journey of a holistic practitioner adapting a business mindset:

- Integrity and Compassion: **Both values emphasize the importance of honesty and ethical practices. For holistic practitioners, this means providing treatments that truly benefit the client, while in business, it reflects fair dealings and transparency. Combining these values ensures that business operations are conducted with the highest ethical standards, fostering trust and loyalty among clients.**
- Resilience and Holism: **The business value of resilience aligns with the holistic principle of treating the whole**

person. Just as resilience encourages bouncing back from setbacks in business, holism involves understanding and addressing the root causes of challenges, whether they are in health or business operations, leading to more sustainable success.

- o Innovation and Continuous Learning: **Innovation in business and continuous learning in holistic practices are about staying ahead through growth and adaptation. Integrating these values encourages the exploration of new healing modalities and business strategies, ensuring the practice remains relevant and impactful.**

- o Determination and Empowerment: **The drive to achieve goals is fundamental in both realms. By adopting determination in their business strategy, holistic practitioners can more effectively empower their clients and themselves, leading to transformative outcomes.**

- o Leadership and Connection: **Effective leadership in business involves inspiring and guiding others toward a shared vision. For holistic practitioners, fostering connections is vital for healing. Combining these aspects enhances the ability to lead a team or** community toward collective wellness and business goals.

o Customer Focus and Mindfulness: Prioritizing customer satisfaction in business aligns with the mindfulness of holistic practices. Both require present, attentive engagement to truly understand and meet the needs of clients, ensuring they receive the utmost value and care.

o Adaptability and Holistic Health Approaches: Being adaptable in business is like embracing various holistic health approaches in practice. Flexibility to change and integrate diverse strategies or treatments can lead to innovative business models that holistically serve both the practitioner and the clientele.

o Philanthropy and Sustainability: The business value of giving back intersects with the holistic value of sustainability. Practitioners who incorporate philanthropy into their business model not only contribute to societal well-being but also reinforce the holistic principle of interconnectivity and care for the environment and community.

By integrating these aligned values, holistic practitioners can cultivate a business mindset that not only drives financial success but also deepens their practice's impact. This harmonious blend enables them to scale their operations while staying true to their core mission of promoting wellness and healing, ultimately achieving a fulfilling and prosperous entrepreneurial journey.

Exercise - Strep 1: Values

- Create a List of Your Values: **Start by listing values that resonate with you deeply. Don't rush this process; take your time to truly connect with what matters most to you.**
- Prioritize: **Once you have a list, prioritize these values based on their significance to you. Which ones are absolutely non-negotiable in how you conduct your business and life?**

Step 2: Uncover Your Motivations

- Personal Motivations: Reflect on what drives you. Is it the desire to heal, to teach, to innovate, or perhaps to build a community? Understanding your personal motivations provides clarity and purpose.
- Journaling: Use a journal to explore these motivations further. Writing can unveil deeper insights into why you're drawn to certain goals or business ideas.

Step 3: Envision the Change You Want

- Visualize Impact: Imagine the ideal outcome of your business efforts. What change do you want to see in your clients, your community, and even globally? Be as detailed as possible in your visualization.
- Create a Vision Board: A vision board can be a powerful tool to keep your desired change visual and front of mind. Include images, quotes, and symbols that represent the impact you aim to achieve.

Step 4: Align Your Business with Your Values and Motivations

- Assessment: Evaluate how your current business model, practices, and offerings align with your identified values and motivations. Where are the gaps, and what feels most aligned?
- Adjustments: Make a plan to adjust aspects of your business that don't fully align with your core values and motivations. This could mean changing how you market your services, the types of services you offer, or even your business operations.

Step 5: Set Goals Based on Desired Change

- SMART Goals: Set Specific, Measurable, Achievable, Relevant, and Time-bound goals that reflect the change you wish to see. Each goal should directly contribute to bringing your vision of change to life.
- Action Plans: For each goal, create a detailed action plan. What steps do you need to take? What resources will you need? Who can support you in achieving these goals?

Step 6: Reflect and Revise Regularly

- Ongoing Reflection: **Make self-reflection a regular part of your routine. As you grow and evolve, so too will your values, motivations, and the change you wish to create.**
- Adapt and Revise: **Be willing to adapt your goals and action plans based on new insights and changes in your personal or business life. The path to realizing your vision is dynamic and requires flexibility.**

Self-reflection is a foundational step in ensuring your business not only succeeds financially but also resonates deeply with your personal values and motivations. By understanding what drives you and the change you want to effect, you can build a business that is truly fulfilling and impactful. This process isn't a one-time task but an ongoing journey of alignment and growth.

Chapter 1 Intentions and Reflective Questions

The Essence of Intent: Understanding and Harnessing Intent for Transformative Success

Intent:

To illuminate the foundational role of intent in driving transformative success, guiding readers to deeply understand and harness their core motivations and aspirations to fuel their holistic practice's growth.

Reflective Questions: *Identifying Your Core Intent*

- What initially drew me to holistic health and entrepreneurship?
- How does this core motivation influence my decisions and direction?

Aligning Intent with Actions:

- In what ways do my current business practices reflect my original intent?
- Are there areas of my practice that feel misaligned with my core motivations, and how can I adjust them?

Intent as a Guiding Force:

- How can I use my intent to navigate challenges and uncertainties in my holistic practice?
- What daily or regular practices can I incorporate to keep my intent clear and at the forefront of my operations?

Measuring Success through Intent:

- Beyond financial metrics, how does my intent help define success for my practice?
- What transformative impacts, both personal and within my client community, do I aim to achieve through my intent?

Evolving Intent:

- As my practice grows and evolves, how might my original intent transform?
- How can I remain open and adaptable to this evolution while staying true to my core values and motivations?

Reflecting on these questions will help you clarify and reinforce your intent, ensuring it serves as a powerful foundation for your holistic practice's growth and success. By understanding and harnessing your intent, you create a purpose-driven path forward, marked by transformation and profound impact.

Chapter 2

From Vision to Reality: Crafting a Vision That Aligns with Your Values and the Greater Good

The Journey from Vision to Reality

Every entrepreneurial venture begins with a vision—a vivid picture of what you aspire to achieve. This vision is more than just an idea; it's a beacon that guides your journey, illuminating the path from where you are now to where you want to be. For holistic health practitioners, crafting a vision that aligns with personal values and the greater good is crucial. It ensures that your business not only thrives financially but also contributes positively to the well-being of individuals and the community.

Crafting Your Vision

- Reflect on Your Core Values: **Your vision should be a true reflection of your deepest beliefs and values. Consider what matters most to you—whether it's healing, sustainability, education, or empowerment— and let these principles guide your vision.**

- Envision the Impact: **Think about the difference you want to make through your business. How do you see your work affecting your clients, the wider community, and even the planet? A compelling vision extends beyond personal success to encompass the well-being of others.**

- Be Specific, Yet Flexible: **While it's important to have a clear and detailed vision, remain open to evolution. As you grow and learn, your vision might expand or shift to incorporate new insights or address emerging needs.**

Aligning Vision with the Greater Good

- Community Engagement: **Connect with your community to understand its needs and how your business can serve them best. This engagement ensures your vision is not only personal but also resonant with those you aim to help.**

- Sustainability Practices: **Incorporate sustainable practices into your business operations, reflecting a commitment to the greater good and setting a precedent in the wellness industry.**

- Education and Advocacy: **Use your platform to educate and advocate for holistic wellness practices, reinforcing the credibility and value of the field.**

Realizing Your Vision

- Strategic Planning: **Break down your vision into actionable goals and steps. A strategic plan acts as a roadmap, turning lofty aspirations into achievable tasks.**

- Gather Resources: **Identify the resources you need— whether it's knowledge, financial investment, or a** supportive network—and actively seek them out. Remember, realizing your vision is a collective effort.

- Embrace the Journey: Be prepared for challenges and setbacks. View these as opportunities for growth and learning. Staying committed to your vision, even when the path gets tough, is what ultimately transforms it into reality.

Transitioning from vision to reality is a dynamic and ongoing process. It requires clarity, commitment, and the courage to dream big. By aligning your vision with your values and the greater good, you create a business that is not only financially successful but also enriching to the soul and beneficial to society. This chapter serves as your guide to infusing your entrepreneurial endeavors with depth, purpose, and transformative potential.

Chapter 2 Intentions and Reflective Questions

From Vision to Reality: Crafting a Vision That Aligns with Your Values and the Greater Good

Intent:

To guide readers in transforming their deep-rooted values and intentions into a clear, actionable vision that not only propels their holistic practice forward but also contributes positively to the greater good.

Reflective Questions: *Defining Your Vision*

- What does my ideal holistic practice look like, and how does it reflect my personal values and the principles of holistic health?

- How does my vision contribute to the greater good, and what specific impacts do I hope to achieve within my community and beyond?

Aligning Vision with Values:

- In what ways do my core values inform my vision for my practice?

- Are there any aspects of my current vision that may not fully align with my values, and how can I adjust them to create harmony?

Translating Vision into Goals:

- What specific, measurable goals can I set that will help bring my vision to reality?

- How can I ensure that these goals not only advance my practice but also uphold my commitment to holistic health and the greater good?

Communicating Your Vision:

- How can I effectively communicate my vision to my clients, team, and broader community to inspire engagement and support?
- What storytelling or messaging strategies can I use to make my vision relatable and compelling?

Evolving Your Vision:

- As my holistic practice grows and the world around me changes, how can I remain open to evolving my vision in response to new insights and needs?
- What practices can I establish to regularly review and refine my vision to ensure it continues to align with my values and the changing landscape of holistic health?

Reflecting on and answering these questions will help you solidify a vision for your holistic practice that is deeply rooted in your values and aspirations for contributing to the greater good. This vision will serve as a north star, guiding your decisions, actions, and growth, ensuring that your practice not only achieves success but also makes a meaningful impact.

PART-2

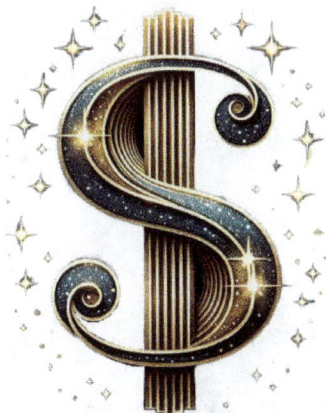

Foundations of

Holistic Business

Growth

Chapter 3

Understanding the Wellness Industry Landscape: Analysis of Current Trends and Opportunities

The Ever-evolving Wellness Industry

The wellness industry is dynamic and expansive, encompassing everything from physical health and nutrition to mental well-being, spirituality, and environmental consciousness. As a holistic practitioner venturing into this industry, it's crucial to grasp its breadth and the trends shaping its future. This understanding will not only ground your business in relevance but also unlock doors to untapped opportunities.

Current Trends in the Wellness Industry

1. Personalization: More than ever, consumers are seeking personalized wellness experiences tailored to their unique health profiles, preferences, and goals. This trend opens opportunities for practitioners to offer customized therapies, programs, and products.

2. Technology Integration: The rise of health and wellness apps, wearable technology, and virtual consultations has transformed how services are delivered and received. Embracing these technologies can expand your reach and enhance your service offerings.

3. Sustainability and Ethical Practices: Consumers are increasingly prioritizing sustainability and ethics in their purchasing decisions. Incorporating eco-friendly practices and ethical sourcing into your business can attract a like-minded clientele.

4. Mental Health Awareness: There's a growing recognition of the importance of mental health alongside physical health. Services that address stress, anxiety, and overall mental well-being are in high demand.

5. Holistic Health Solutions: **The shift toward holistic health solutions, which consider the entire individual rather than just symptoms, is gaining momentum. This trend aligns perfectly with the holistic practitioner's approach.**

Identifying Opportunities

- Market Research: **Conduct thorough research to identify gaps in the market that your business can fill. Look for underserved areas within the holistic wellness space where your unique skills and knowledge can make a difference.**
- Networking: **Engage with industry peers, attend wellness conferences, and participate in online forums to stay informed about emerging trends and opportunities.**
- Customer Feedback: **Listen to your clients. Their needs and interests can guide you toward new areas for business expansion or improvement.**

Leveraging Trends for Business Growth

- Innovation: Use your understanding of current trends to innovate your offerings. Whether it's through incorporating new healing modalities, adopting green business practices, or offering online consultations, staying ahead of trends can set your business apart.

- Education and Communication: Educate your audience about the benefits of holistic health practices and how your services align with current trends. Effective communication can position you as a thought leader in your field.

Grasping the wellness industry landscape is foundational for any holistic business aiming to grow and thrive. By understanding current trends and identifying opportunities, you can strategically position your business to meet the evolving needs of your clients and the broader community. This chapter equips you with the knowledge to navigate the industry's complexities, ensuring your holistic practice not only survives but flourishes in this dynamic environment.

Step-by-Step Action for Market Research

Step 1: Define Your Objectives

- Start by clearly defining what you hope to achieve with your market research. Are you looking to expand your service offerings, enter a new market, or understand your competition better?

Step 2: Gather Preliminary Information

- Begin with a broad overview of the wellness industry. Use online resources, industry reports, and publications to get a sense of current trends and the competitive landscape.

Step 3: Identify Your Niche

- Narrow down your focus to the specific areas of holistic wellness that align with your expertise and passion. This could be anything from nutritional counseling to stress management techniques.

Step 4: Analyze the Competition

- Identify other businesses offering similar services. Note what they do well and where there might be gaps in their offerings. This can highlight opportunities for differentiation.

Step 5: Understand Your Target Audience

Define who your ideal clients are. Consider factors such as age, lifestyle, health concerns, and where they seek wellness information. Surveys, interviews, and social media can provide insights into their needs and preferences.

Step 6: Identify Gaps and Opportunities

Based on your understanding of the market and your target audience, identify gaps in the market. These are areas where customer needs are not fully met by current offerings.

Step 7: Evaluate Your Findings

Take a step back and evaluate the information you've gathered. Look for clear signs of demand that align with your skills and the unique value you can offer.

Step 8: Validate Your Ideas

Before fully committing to a new direction, seek validation. This could be through pilot programs, offering free trials, or getting feedback from a small group of trusted clients.

Step 9: Develop a Plan

With validated ideas in hand, develop a strategic plan to fill the identified market gaps. This should include service development, marketing strategies, and any necessary training or certification you might need.

Step 10: Implement and Monitor

Put your plan into action. As you roll out new services or enter new markets, closely monitor client feedback and business performance. Be prepared to make adjustments based on what you learn.

Market research is a critical step in identifying opportunities for growth in the holistic wellness space. By systematically gathering and analyzing information, you can make informed decisions that align with your expertise and meet the needs of your target audience, setting your business up for success.

Example for Each of the 10 Market Research Steps

Step 1: Define Your Objectives

- Objective: To explore the potential for integrating yoga therapy into a holistic nutrition counseling service.

Step 2: Gather Preliminary Information

- Action: Read recent industry reports on the growth of yoga therapy and holistic nutrition. Visit forums and social media groups focused on holistic health trends.

Step 3: Identify Your Niche

- Niche Focus: Combining yoga therapy with nutritional counseling for clients dealing with stress and anxiety.

Step 4: Analyze the Competition

- Action: Identify three local wellness centers offering yoga or nutrition counseling. Note that none offer a combined service specifically targeted at stress and anxiety relief.

Step 5: Understand Your Target Audience

- Target Audience: Adults aged 25-45, experiencing stress and anxiety, interested in holistic wellness practices but new to yoga and nutrition counseling.

Step 6: Identify Gaps and Opportunities

- Identified Gap: Lack of integrated services that combine yoga with personalized nutrition plans for stress relief.

Step 7: Evaluate Your Findings

- Evaluation: There's a growing interest in holistic approaches to managing stress and anxiety. However, current offerings are fragmented, indicating an opportunity for an integrated service.

Step 8: Validate Your Ideas

- Validation: Offer a free introductory workshop on "Yoga and Nutrition for Stress Relief" to gauge interest and collect feedback from participants.

Step 9: Develop a Plan

- Plan: Create a 6-week program combining weekly yoga sessions with personalized nutrition counseling, targeted at individuals seeking natural ways to manage stress and anxiety.

Step 10: Implement and Monitor

- Implementation: Launch the program with an initial cohort, promoting it through social media, local wellness fairs, and partnerships with mental health professionals. Collect participant feedback weekly to adjust the program as needed.

This example illustrates a step-by-step approach to market research, from identifying a potential opportunity in integrating yoga therapy into holistic nutrition counseling to implementing and monitoring a new program. Each step builds on the previous one, ensuring the decision to launch a new service is informed, targeted, and responsive to client needs.

Chapter 3 Intentions and Reflective Questions

Understanding the Wellness Industry Landscape: Analysis of Current Trends and Opportunities

Intent:

To equip readers with the knowledge to navigate the dynamic wellness industry landscape, Identifying current trends and uncovering opportunities that align with their holistic practice's mission and vision.

Reflective Questions: *Industry Trends Analysis:*

- Which current trends in the wellness industry resonate with my holistic practice's values and offerings?
- How can I stay informed about emerging trends and adapt my practice to remain relevant and responsive?

Opportunity Identification:

- What gaps or unmet needs exist in the current wellness industry that my practice could address?
- How can I leverage my unique skills and insights to create offerings that fill these gaps?

Competitive Landscape:

- Who are my main competitors within the holistic wellness space, and what can I learn from their successes and challenges?
- How does my practice differentiate itself from competitors, and how can I communicate this unique value proposition to my target audience?

Consumer Needs and Preferences:

- What are the changing needs and preferences of wellness consumers, and how can my practice evolve to meet these demands?

- How can I engage with my clients and community to gain deeper insights into their wellness journeys and how my practice can support them?

Sustainability and Ethical Practices:

- How are sustainability and ethical practices influencing the wellness industry, and how can my practice incorporate these values?

- What steps can I take to ensure my practice not only contributes to individual well-being but also to the well-being of the planet and society at large?

Technological Advancements:

- What role do technological advancements play in the wellness industry, and how can my practice harness technology to enhance service delivery and client engagement?

- Are there specific technologies or digital platforms that could elevate my practice's offerings and accessibility?

Reflecting upon these questions allows you to critically assess the wellness industry landscape, recognizing trends that align with your holistic practice. This understanding enables you to strategically position your practice to seize opportunities, differentiate from competitors, and meet the evolving needs of your clients, ensuring long-term growth and impact in the wellness domain.

Chapter 4

Elevating and Expanding Your Holistic Practice: A Blueprint for New and Established Practitioners

Crafting a Vision That Grows with You

Whether you're laying the groundwork for a new venture or seeking to scale an established practice, the first step is to articulate a vision that encapsulates your holistic ethos while embracing ambitious growth. This vision should reflect a commitment to enhancing well-being on all levels—personal, communal, and environmental—and adapt as your business evolves.

Service Innovation: Meeting Needs at Every Scale

- **For New Practitioners:** Focus on identifying niche services that align with your unique skills and the specific needs of your target audience. This might mean offering personalized wellness coaching or specialized treatments that set you apart.

- **For Established Practitioners:** Look into diversifying your offerings with scalable options like online workshops, digital products, or group programs that allow you to reach a wider audience without diluting the personalized care that defines your practice.

Creating Holistic Experiences That Resonate

- Design client experiences that reinforce your holistic values, from the initial consultation through ongoing engagement. Utilize technology to maintain a personal touch as you grow, ensuring every interaction is meaningful and supports the client's journey toward holistic well-being.

Fostering a Vibrant Community

- Building a supportive community is essential, whether you're just starting out or aiming to broaden your practice's impact. Engage with your audience through social media, collaborative events, and wellness forums. For established businesses, consider creating ambassador programs or client success stories to deepen connections and attract new clients.

Sustainability: A Core Principle of Growth

- Embed sustainability into your business model from day one. This commitment should influence everything from your operational choices to your service offerings, ensuring that as your business grows, it does so in a way that benefits the planet and its inhabitants.

Leading by Example

- Your personal commitment to holistic well-being is your practice's heart and soul. Share your journey, practices, and the lessons learned along the way. This authenticity will inspire trust and loyalty among your clients, regardless of your business's size.

Mindfully Integrating Technology

- Evaluate and integrate technologies that complement your holistic approach. For new practitioners, simple tools like scheduling software or virtual consultation platforms can enhance efficiency. Established businesses might explore developing custom wellness apps or leveraging AI for personalized wellness recommendations.

Empowering Through Holistic Education

- Education is a powerful tool for empowerment. Offer workshops, create content, or even write articles that help demystify holistic health practices. As your practice grows, consider launching online courses or speaking at events to share your knowledge more broadly.

Redefining Success on Your Terms

- Success in a holistic business isn't just measured by financial milestones but by the positive impact on clients' lives, community well-being, and environmental sustainability. Set holistic KPIs that reflect these dimensions, ensuring your growth enriches both your practice and the broader ecosystem.

Whether you're just stepping into the world of holistic health or are looking to scale an existing practice, the journey ahead is rich with opportunities to make a profound impact. By grounding your business in holistic principles, embracing innovation, and committing to sustainability, you can create a practice that not only thrives financially but also fosters true well-being for your clients and the planet. This blueprint is your guide to navigating the challenges and opportunities of growing a holistic practice in today's dynamic wellness landscape.

Chapter 4 Intentions and Reflective Questions

Elevating and Expanding Your Holistic Practice: A Blueprint for New and Established Practitioners

Intent:

To provide both new and seasoned holistic practitioners with a strategic blueprint for elevating and expanding their practice, focusing on actionable steps that enhance service quality, client satisfaction, and business growth.

Reflective Questions: *Assessing Your Current Position*

- Where does my practice currently stand in terms of client base, service offerings, and market positioning?
- What are the strengths of my practice, and where do I see opportunities for improvement and expansion?

Setting Growth Objectives:

- What specific objectives do I have for growing my practice in the short term (1-2 years) and long term (5 years and beyond)?
- How do these objectives align with my overall vision for my practice and the impact I want to make in the holistic health field?

Enhancing Service Offerings:

- How can I enhance or diversify my current services to better meet the needs of my clients and attract new ones?
- Are there new or emerging holistic practices or technologies that I can integrate into my offerings to provide added value?

Building a Strong Community Presence:

- What strategies can I employ to strengthen my practice's presence within my local community and beyond?
- How can community engagement and partnerships contribute to the growth and visibility of my practice?

Leveraging Digital Marketing and Online Platforms:

- How effectively am I using digital marketing and online platforms to reach my target audience and promote my services?
- What improvements or new tactics can I implement to enhance my online presence and attract a wider audience?

Professional Development and Networking:

- In what ways can I continue to develop professionally to ensure that I remain at the forefront of the holistic health field?

- How can networking with other holistic health professionals and joining professional associations support my practice's growth?

Client Retention and Satisfaction:

- How do I currently measure client satisfaction, and what feedback mechanisms are in place to gather insights from my clients?
- What strategies can I introduce to improve client retention and ensure that clients have a positive and transformative experience with my practice?

Operational Efficiency and Scalability:

- What operational challenges am I facing, and how can I streamline processes to improve efficiency?
- As I plan for expansion, what considerations should I take into account to ensure that my practice can scale effectively?

Reflecting on these questions provides a comprehensive framework for critically evaluating your holistic practice from various angles—service quality, client engagement, market presence, and operational efficiency. This blueprint encourages both new and established practitioners to adopt a strategic approach to growth, ensuring their practice not only thrives financially but also continues to make a significant impact on the well-being of their clients and community.

Chapter 5

Building a Business on Holistic Principles: Integrating Holistic Practices into Your Business Model for Sustained Success

The Foundation of Holistic Business

At the core of a holistic business model lies the commitment to treating individuals and communities as interconnected wholes, recognizing that all aspects of one's environment, body, mind, and spirit influence well-being. This chapter guides you through integrating these holistic principles into your business model, creating a foundation not just for financial success but for making a profound, positive impact.

Step 1: Define Your Holistic Vision

- Craft a Vision Statement: Your vision should encapsulate the holistic impact you aim to achieve through your business. For example, "To empower individuals to achieve optimal well-being by integrating body, mind, and spirit into our wellness programs."

Step 2: Align Services with Holistic Values

- Service Design: Ensure each service or product you offer aligns with holistic principles. If you're a nutritional therapist, for instance, this might mean incorporating mindfulness practices into your dietary plans, acknowledging the mental and emotional components of eating.

Step 3: Create a Holistic Client Experience

- Client Journey: Design the client experience from first contact through ongoing engagement to reflect holistic values. This could involve comprehensive assessments that consider all aspects of a client's life and personalized follow-ups that support their entire well-being journey.

Step 4: Foster a Supportive Community

- Build Community: A holistic business thrives on the strength of its community. Host workshops, retreats, or online forums that bring clients together, not just as consumers of a service but as participants in a shared journey toward wellness.

Step 5: Commit to Sustainability

- Eco-friendly Practices: Your business operations should mirror the holistic respect for the environment. Use sustainable materials, reduce waste, and consider the ecological footprint of your products and services.

Step 6: Practice What You Preach

- Personal Well-being: As a holistic entrepreneur, your own health and wellness are paramount. Lead by example, showing clients and employees alike that holistic well-being is at the heart of your business's success.

Step 7: Leverage Technology Responsibly

- Tech for Holism: Use technology to enhance, not detract from, the holistic nature of your services. This might involve digital platforms that facilitate meditation sessions or apps that help clients track their holistic health progress.

Step 8: Educate and Empower

- Holistic Education: Beyond providing services, educate your clients on holistic principles. This empowerment helps them make informed choices about their health and wellness, extending the impact of your work.

Step 9: Measure Success Holistically

- Beyond Financial Metrics: While financial growth is important, also measure success in terms of client well-being, community impact, and environmental sustainability. These metrics ensure your business remains true to its holistic roots as it scales.

Integrating holistic practices into your business model isn't just about offering a range of services; it's about weaving a commitment to comprehensive well-being into every aspect of your business, from how you interact with clients to how you operate behind the scenes. By building your business on these principles, you create a model that is not only financially successful but also profoundly transformative for your clients and the wider community, truly scaling beyond six figures in every sense of the term.

Chapter 5 Intentions and Reflective Questions

Building a Business on Holistic Principles: Integrating Holistic Practices into Your Business Model for Sustained Success

Intent:

To guide readers in embedding holistic principles deeply within their business models, ensuring that every aspect of their operation reflects a commitment to holistic health, sustainability, and ethical practices for long-lasting success.

Reflective Questions: *Defining Holistic Principles in Business*

- What do holistic principles mean to me personally, and how do they translate into my business practices?
- How can I ensure my business operations, from sourcing to service delivery, align with these holistic principles?

Holistic Product/Service Development:

- In developing new products or services, how can I incorporate holistic health principles to enhance client well-being?
- What checks and balances can I put in place to ensure my offerings remain true to holistic ethics over time?

Sustainability and Environmental Responsibility:

- How does my business currently impact the environment, and what steps can I take to minimize my ecological footprint?
- In what ways can I promote sustainability within my practice and encourage my clients to adopt environmentally responsible behaviors?

Client Relationships and Community Engagement:

- How can I foster deeper, more holistic relationships with my clients that go beyond transactional interactions?
- What role can my business play in supporting and nurturing the wider community's health and wellness?

Employee Well-being and Workplace Culture:

- How can I create a workplace culture that reflects holistic principles and supports the well-being of my team?
- What practices or policies can I implement to ensure my employees feel valued, supported, and motivated?

Ethical Marketing and Communication:

- How can I ensure my marketing strategies and communications are transparent, honest, and reflective of my holistic values?
- What methods can I use to educate my audience about the benefits of holistic health practices without resorting to misleading claims?

Financial Integrity and Pricing Models:

- How can I develop pricing models and financial strategies that are fair, transparent, and allow for the accessibility of my services to a broader audience?
- What measures can I take to ensure financial decisions are made with integrity, prioritizing client welfare and community benefit?

Continuous Learning and Adaptation:

- How can I stay informed about advancements in holistic health practices and integrate relevant findings into my business?
- What processes can I establish to regularly review and refine my business model in alignment with evolving holistic principles?

Reflecting on these questions encourages a holistic approach to every aspect of running a health and wellness business. It challenges practitioners to not only consider the direct impact of their services but also the broader implications of their business decisions on the environment, community, and internal team dynamics. By deeply integrating holistic principles into your business model, you create a practice that not only achieves sustained success but also contributes positively to the collective well-being.

Chapter 6

Strategic Planning and Scaling: Key Strategies for Growth and Expansion in the Holistic Wellness Sector

Whether you're dreaming of launching a holistic wellness practice or you're ready to take your existing business to new heights, understanding the art of strategic planning and scaling is crucial. This chapter unveils key strategies designed to help you surpass the six-figure mark, focusing on growth and expansion while staying true to the heart of holistic wellness.

1. Define Your Unique Value Proposition (UVP)

- What Makes You Different: **Begin by clearly articulating what sets your holistic wellness practice apart from others. Your UVP should highlight your unique approach, specialized services, or the particular health** outcomes your clients can expect. Knowing this will guide all your scaling efforts, ensuring you stand out in a crowded market.

2. Diversify Your Service Offerings

- Expand Mindfully: Consider broadening your range of services to address different aspects of holistic wellness, such as adding complementary therapies, group sessions, or online courses. Diversification should be done thoughtfully, ensuring each new offering aligns with your core mission and meets a clear client need.

3. Embrace Digital Transformation

- Leverage Technology: Utilize digital platforms to extend your reach. This could mean offering virtual consultations, creating a wellness app, or launching an online learning platform. Digital solutions can help you scale your impact without being limited by physical location or capacity.

4. Build Strategic Partnerships

- Collaborate for Growth: Partnering with other businesses or practitioners can open up new opportunities. Look for synergies with non-competing services in the wellness space, such as fitness centers, health food stores, or mental health professionals. Together, you can offer more comprehensive wellness solutions and tap into each other's client bases.

5. Optimize Operational Efficiency

- Streamline Processes: As your business grows, maintaining operational efficiency becomes essential. Invest in systems and software that automate routine tasks, from scheduling appointments to managing client records. This frees up time to focus on scaling efforts and enhancing client experiences.

6. Focus on Client Retention and Referrals

- Cultivate Loyalty: Happy clients are your best advocates. Implement loyalty programs, offer exclusive content, or create a referral incentive scheme.

Fostering a strong, engaged client community not only supports retention but can also attract new clients through word-of-mouth.

7. Invest in Your Online Presence

- Digital Marketing: A robust online presence can significantly boost your visibility. Invest in a professional website, engage on social media platforms where your target clients are active, and consider content marketing to establish your expertise in the holistic wellness field.

8. Continuous Learning and Innovation

- Stay Ahead of Trends: The wellness industry is constantly evolving. Keep learning and adapting your offerings based on the latest research, client feedback, and industry trends. Staying innovative ensures your practice remains relevant and competitive.

9. Financial Planning and Management

- Smart Financial Strategies: Understand your numbers. Regularly review your financial performance, set clear revenue goals, and manage cash flow carefully. Consider working with a financial advisor to explore investment opportunities or funding options to fuel growth.

10. Measure, Analyze, and Adjust

- Adapt Based on Insights: Use data and feedback to continually refine your strategies. Tracking key performance indicators (KPIs) will help you understand what's working and where adjustments are needed, ensuring your scaling efforts are effective and aligned with your goals.

Scaling beyond six figures in the holistic wellness sector requires a combination of strategic thinking, operational excellence, and a deep commitment to your core values. By implementing these key strategies, you can expand your impact, reach a wider audience, and achieve financial success without losing sight of the holistic principles that define your practice. Welcome to the next level of your entrepreneurial journey in wellness.

Chapter 6 Intentions and Reflective Questions

Strategic Planning and Scaling: Key Strategies for Growth and Expansion in the Holistic Wellness Sector

Intent:

To empower holistic wellness professionals with strategic insights and methodologies for planning and executing growth initiatives, ensuring their practice scales effectively and sustainably within the holistic wellness sector.

Reflective Questions: *Assessing Readiness for Scaling*

- What indicators suggest my practice is ready for scaling, and what areas might need strengthening before expansion?
- How does my current operational capacity match up with my aspirations for growth?

Defining Your Growth Strategy:

- What specific areas of my practice offer the greatest potential for growth (e.g., expanding service offerings, entering new markets, leveraging technology)?
- How can I ensure that my growth strategy aligns with my holistic principles and the long-term vision for my practice?

Understanding Market Dynamics:

- How do current trends in the holistic wellness sector influence my opportunities for expansion?
- What market research can I conduct or refer to for deeper insights into potential growth areas?

Developing a Scalable Business Model:

- What changes or adjustments to my business model are necessary to support sustainable scaling?
- How can I structure my practice to maintain quality and personalization of services as I grow?

Financial Planning for Expansion:

- What financial resources will I need to support my growth strategy, and what are my options for securing these funds?
- How will I measure the financial success of my scaling efforts, and what benchmarks should I set?

Building and Managing a Growing Team:

- What roles and skills will be essential in my expanded practice, and how can I attract and retain talent that aligns with my holistic mission?
- How can I maintain a cohesive team culture and ensure that all team members are committed to our shared holistic values as we grow?

Innovating and Diversifying Offerings:

- What innovative services or products can I introduce to differentiate my practice in a competitive market?
- How can I involve my clients in the innovation process to ensure new offerings meet their needs and expectations?

Maintaining Quality and Integrity During Growth:

- What measures and systems can I put in place to ensure that the quality of care and adherence to holistic principles do not diminish as my practice expands?
- How will I balance the need for operational efficiency with the personal touch and individualized care that define holistic wellness?

Reflecting on these questions enables holistic wellness professionals to approach strategic planning and scaling with a clear, informed perspective. By carefully considering each aspect of growth, from readiness assessment to quality maintenance, you can expand your practice in a way that not only increases its reach and profitability but also deepens its impact and upholds its commitment to holistic health and well-being.

PART-3

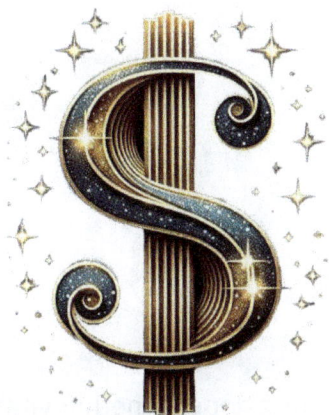

Strategies for

Scaling Beyond

Six Figures

Chapter 7

Financial Mastery in Wellness: Navigating Finances, Investments, and Revenue Streams for Holistic Businesses

As a holistic health practitioner, whether you're just embarking on your entrepreneurial journey or seeking to elevate an existing practice, mastering the financial aspects of your business is crucial. This chapter delves into financial mastery within the wellness industry, offering insights on managing finances, exploring investment opportunities, and diversifying revenue streams to ensure your holistic business not only thrives but flourishes financially.

1. Understanding Financial Basics

- Financial Literacy: Begin by ensuring you have a solid understanding of financial basics, including accounting, budgeting, and financial planning. Familiarize yourself with key financial statements like the balance sheet, income statement, and cash flow statement. This knowledge is crucial for making informed decisions.

2. Setting Up Financial Systems

- **Efficient Systems:** Implement accounting software tailored to small businesses to track your income and expenses accurately. Consider hiring a professional accountant or bookkeeper who can offer tailored advice and ensure you're compliant with tax laws.

3. Budgeting for Growth

- **Create a Budget:** Develop a comprehensive budget that accounts for all aspects of your business operations, from rent and utilities to marketing and staff salaries. Regularly review and adjust your budget to reflect actual spending and shifting priorities.

4. Exploring Investment Opportunities

- **Investment for Expansion:** Look into various investment options to support your business growth.

This could include taking out a business loan, seeking out angel investors, or exploring government grants for small businesses in the wellness sector.

5. Diversifying Revenue Streams

- Broaden Your Offerings: **Diversify your income by adding new services, products, or even passive income streams such as online courses, wellness products, or membership programs. Each additional stream can help stabilize your income and reduce financial risk.**

6. Pricing Strategies

- Value-Based Pricing: **Develop pricing strategies that reflect the value and results your services offer, rather than simply competing on price. This might mean setting higher prices for specialized services or offering packages that provide more comprehensive support.**
- To achieve a six-figure income ($100,000) annually with five clients per day at $100 each:
    - Per Session: $100
    - Per Day (5 clients): $100 x 5 = $500
    - Per Week (5 days): $500 x 5 = $2,500

- o Per Month: To achieve $100,000 annually, you would divide by 12, equating to approximately $8,333.33 per month.
  - o Per Year: $100,000
- To scale up to a seven-figure income ($1,000,000) annually under the same conditions:
  - o Per Day (5 clients): Still $500, as the session price remains constant.
  - o Per Week (5 days): To reach a seven-figure income, you'd need to increase either the number of clients or the price per session, or work more weeks. But at the base rate of $500 per day, it's about scaling operations.
  - o Per Month: Dividing $1,000,000 by 12 months, you would need to make approximately $83,333.33 per month.
  - o Per Year: $1,000,000

To realistically achieve these figures, consider:

- Increasing the number of daily clients or sessions.
- Raising your rates based on the value you provide.

- Expanding your offerings to include packages, group sessions, workshops, or online courses for additional revenue streams.
- Implementing passive income strategies, such as digital products or memberships.

Remember, achieving these income goals requires not just hard work but also strategic planning, financial management, and possibly expanding your team or resources to handle the increased workload and broaden your business's impact.

7. Managing Cash Flow

- Cash Flow Management: Keep a close eye on your cash flow—the lifeblood of your business. Effective cash flow management ensures you can cover your operational costs and invest in growth opportunities without stretching your finances too thin.

8. Planning for Taxes

- Tax Strategy: Plan ahead for taxes to avoid any surprises. Work with a tax professional to identify potential deductions and credits related to your holistic business and strategize for efficient tax planning.

9. Saving and Investing for the Future

- Future Financial Security: **Set aside a portion of your profits for savings and investments, securing not only your business's future but also your personal financial well-being.**

10. Analyzing Financial Performance

- Performance Review: **Regularly analyze your financial performance to identify trends, opportunities for cost savings, and areas for revenue growth. Use this analysis to refine your financial strategy and ensure sustainable business growth.**

Achieving financial mastery in wellness requires a blend of practical financial management, strategic planning, and a commitment to your holistic principles. By navigating your finances wisely, exploring investments, and diversifying your revenue streams, you can build a financially robust holistic business poised for long-term success and impact. Remember, financial health is an integral part of your holistic business's overall well-being, enabling you to serve your clients and community more effectively.

FOR THE EXPERIENCED HOLISTIC ENTREPRENEUR

For someone who already owns a holistic business and is seeking ways to scale, focusing on advanced financial strategies becomes crucial. Here are key points tailored to your situation:

1. Financial Analysis for Scaling: **Dive deep into your current financial statements to identify trends, profitability by service or product, and areas of inefficiency. This analysis can reveal where to focus your scaling efforts for maximum impact.**

2. Revisiting and Refining Your Pricing Model: **As you scale, your pricing strategy may need adjustments. Consider value-based pricing to better reflect the outcomes and transformations your services provide. This could mean introducing premium packages or memberships that offer more comprehensive solutions.**

3. Advanced Budgeting Techniques: **Employ more sophisticated budgeting, forecasting future income and expenses with scaling in mind. Incorporate scenarios for expansion, such as hiring staff, investing in marketing, or opening new locations, and how these will impact your financials.**

4. Securing Growth Capital: **If scaling your operations requires significant upfront investment, explore options for securing growth capital. This could include business loans, investor funding, or strategic partnerships that provide both capital and expansion opportunities.**

5. Optimizing Cash Flow Management: **For a scaling business, managing cash flow becomes even more critical. Implement strategies to improve cash flow, such as tightening credit terms, optimizing inventory, or leveraging payment plans for clients.**

6. Financial Metrics and KPIs for Scaling: **Establish financial Key Performance Indicators (KPIs) specific to scaling objectives. These might include customer acquisition cost, lifetime value, profit margins by service line, and return on investment for marketing campaigns.**

7. Tax Planning for Growth: Anticipate how scaling will affect your tax situation. Proactive tax planning can help minimize liabilities and take advantage of credits or deductions available for business expansion activities.

8. Scaling with Financial Sustainability in Mind: Ensure your scaling efforts are financially sustainable. This means not just chasing growth for growth's sake but focusing on profitable, manageable expansion that aligns with your long-term business goals and values.

9. Exploring Exit Strategies or Succession Planning: As part of your scaling strategy, consider your long-term goals for the business, including potential exit strategies or succession planning. Understanding these options can influence financial planning and business structuring decisions.

10. Continuous Financial Education: As your business grows, so too will the complexity of its financial needs. Commit to ongoing learning about financial management, investments, and economic trends that could impact your business.

Scaling a holistic business requires not just passion and expertise in your field but also sophisticated financial management. By focusing on these advanced strategies, you can ensure your business not only grows in size but also in financial health, stability, and impact.

Chapter 7 Intentions and Reflective Questions

Financial Mastery in Wellness: Navigating Finances, Investments, and Revenue Streams for Holistic Businesses

Intent:

To guide holistic health professionals in mastering the financial aspects of their business, from managing day-to-day finances and exploring investment opportunities to diversifying revenue streams, ensuring financial health and sustainability.

Reflective Questions: *Understanding Financial Health*

- What are the key financial metrics I should regularly monitor to ensure the health of my holistic practice?
- How can I improve my financial literacy to make informed decisions that align with both my business and holistic values?

Investment Strategies:

- What types of investments are suitable for a holistic business looking to grow sustainably?
- How can I attract investors who share my vision for holistic wellness and understand the unique value of my practice?

Diversifying Revenue Streams:

- What potential revenue streams have I not yet explored that could align with and enhance my holistic practice?
- How can I innovate my service offerings or create products that meet my clients' needs while also contributing to steady revenue growth?

Budgeting and Financial Planning:

- How can I create a budget that accounts for both the operational needs of my practice and my goals for expansion?
- What tools or resources can assist me in planning and tracking my finances more effectively?

Managing Expenses:

- How can I evaluate my current expenses to identify areas where I can reduce costs without compromising the quality of care or service?
- What strategies can I implement to manage cash flow effectively, especially during slower business periods?

Pricing Models:

- How do I develop pricing models for my services and products that reflect their value, support my financial goals, and remain accessible to my target clientele?
- What considerations should I take into account when adjusting prices in response to costs, competition, or market demand?

Funding and Grants for Holistic Practices:

- What sources of funding or grants are available specifically for holistic health businesses, and how can I access them?
- How do I prepare a compelling application for funding that highlights the impact and potential of my holistic practice?

Financial Ethics in Holistic Health:

- How can I ensure that my financial practices reflect ethical considerations, transparency, and fairness to my clients and community?
- What measures can I put in place to protect client information and financial data in accordance with best practices and regulations?

Reflecting on these questions empowers holistic health professionals to take charge of the financial aspects of their business confidently. Financial mastery is not just about ensuring profitability but about fostering a business environment where holistic principles, ethical practices, and financial sustainability coexist harmoniously, allowing you to continue making a positive impact through your work.

Chapter 8

Marketing with Authenticity: Effective Branding and Marketing Strategies That Resonate with Your Core Audience

In the holistic wellness industry, authenticity isn't just a buzzword—it's the foundation of effective marketing and branding. Whether you're just starting your holistic practice or are an experienced practitioner aiming to scale, connecting genuinely with your audience is key to building trust and loyalty. This chapter explores how to craft and implement marketing strategies that reflect your true self and speak directly to the hearts of your clients.

1. Define Your Authentic Brand

Discover Your Brand Voice: Your brand voice is an authentic expression of your values, beliefs, and the unique approach you bring to wellness. It should be consistent across all marketing materials, from your website to social media posts.

Visual Identity: Create a visual identity that reflects the essence of your practice. Use colors, fonts, and imagery that convey the feelings of calm, healing, and wellness you want clients to associate with your brand.

2. Tell Your Story

Share Your Journey: People love stories, especially those that inspire or resonate with their own experiences. Share your journey into holistic wellness, including the challenges you've overcome and the successes you've celebrated. This not only humanizes your brand but also builds a deeper connection with your audience.

3. Content Marketing

Educate and Inspire: Use your blog, videos, and social media to share valuable content that educates and inspires your audience. Topics could range from wellness tips and success stories to insights into holistic practices. Quality, valuable content can position you as an authority in your field.

4. Social Media Engagement

Genuine Interaction: Use social media platforms not just to broadcast but to engage in meaningful conversations with your community. Respond to comments, ask for feedback, and participate in relevant discussions. Authentic engagement enhances your visibility and credibility.

5. Email Marketing

Personalized Communication: Email newsletters are a powerful tool for maintaining connection with your clients. Share updates, exclusive content, or personalized wellness tips. Segment your email list to ensure the content is relevant and engaging for different groups within your audience.

6. Collaborations and Partnerships

Align with Like-minded Brands: Collaborate with other businesses or practitioners who share your holistic values. This could be through joint workshops, cross-promotions, or shared content. Such partnerships can introduce your brand to new audiences while reinforcing your authentic commitment to wellness.

7. Client Testimonials and Success Stories

Leverage Social Proof: Positive experiences and transformations are compelling. Encourage satisfied clients to share their stories through testimonials or case studies. These real-life endorsements serve as powerful social proof, validating the effectiveness of your holistic approach.

8. Community Involvement

- Give Back: Participate in community wellness events or host free workshops. Giving back not only demonstrates your commitment to holistic well-being beyond profit but also strengthens your local presence and network.

Marketing with authenticity is about more than just selling your services; it's about creating genuine connections and building a community around shared values of wellness and transformation. By integrating these strategies into your holistic practice, you attract and retain clients who not only believe in what you do but are also eager to support and advocate for your brand. Remember, in the world of holistic wellness, your authenticity is your most potent marketing tool.

Marketing with Authenticity: A Success Story

Meet Ava: Ava, a certified holistic nutritionist, embarked on her journey driven by a personal battle with chronic health issues. Through holistic practices, she not only transformed her health but discovered a passion for helping others achieve wellness. Determined to share her insights and solutions, Ava launched "Nourish & Flourish," a holistic nutrition counseling service.

Defining the Brand: Ava began by crafting a brand that was a true reflection of her journey and values. She chose a serene color palette that mirrored the calm and healing she wanted her clients to feel. Her logo, a sprouting seed, symbolized growth and transformation. Ava's brand voice was warm, encouraging, and rooted in her genuine desire to support others on their wellness journey.

Telling Her Story: **Recognizing the power of storytelling, Ava** shared her wellness journey on her website and social media, detailing the struggles she faced and the holistic practices that turned her life around. This personal narrative resonated deeply with her audience, many of whom saw reflections of their own struggles in Ava's story.

Engaging Content Marketing: **Ava regularly published blog** posts and videos offering valuable nutrition advice, wellness tips, and client success stories. Her content was not only informative but also inspirational, showcasing real-life examples of transformation through holistic nutrition.

Social Media Engagement: **On social media, Ava didn't just** post and disappear. She engaged actively with her followers, answering their questions, celebrating their successes, and creating a sense of community. She hosted live Q&A sessions, where she shared her expertise and connected with her audience on a personal level.

Personalized Email Marketing: **Ava's email newsletters were a** hit. She segmented her email list to offer personalized tips and updates, making her clients feel seen and understood. Her emails often included invitations to free workshops, emphasizing her commitment to providing value beyond her paid services.

Collaborations for Greater Reach: Ava partnered with a local yoga studio to offer a "Wellness Weekend" retreat, combining yoga with holistic nutrition workshops. This collaboration not only introduced her services to a new audience but also highlighted her holistic approach to wellness, aligning perfectly with her brand.

Leveraging Client Testimonials: Satisfied clients were eager to share their stories, thanks to Ava's encouragement. These testimonials were featured on her website and social media, providing powerful social proof of her service's effectiveness.

Community Involvement: Ava frequently volunteered at community health fairs, offering free nutrition consultations. This not only cemented her reputation as a knowledgeable and caring practitioner but also aligned with her brand's mission of accessible wellness for all.

The Outcome: "Nourish & Flourish" thrived, distinguished by a brand that was genuinely Ava's. Her authentic marketing approach attracted clients who were not just looking for nutrition advice but sought transformation guided by someone who had walked the path before them. Ava's story illustrates that marketing with authenticity isn't just effective; it's transformative—for both the business and its clients.

As Ava watched "Nourish & Flourish" flourish, she dreamed bigger, setting her sights on a seven-figure horizon. But scaling to such heights was more than just a financial goal; it was about extending her impact, touching more lives globally while staying true to the essence that had defined her success: authenticity and deep, personal connections. Here's how Ava embraced this ambitious journey, transforming her dream into a blueprint for holistic growth.

Digital Frontiers: Expanding Reach: Ava ventured into digital offerings, developing an online course that distilled her holistic nutrition expertise into an accessible format. This wasn't just a course; it was an invitation to wellness, complete with video lessons, downloadable resources, and live interactions, allowing Ava to extend her nurturing guidance worldwide.

Building a Community: Membership and More: To deepen connections, Ava introduced a membership program, "The

Wellness Circle." It was a digital sanctuary offering exclusive content, personalized plans, and a supportive community. This recurring model didn't just ensure steady revenue; it fostered a tight-knit community, bonded by shared wellness journeys.

Team Nourish & Flourish: Strategic Hiring: Recognizing the limits of solo scaling, Ava built a team of experts. Nutritionists, wellness coaches, and content creators joined her mission, enabling "Nourish & Flourish" to offer a broader spectrum of services without diluting the quality that had become its hallmark.

Authenticity in Marketing: Touching Hearts Worldwide: Ava harnessed the power of paid advertising and authentic influencer partnerships to expand her audience. These efforts were grounded in her unique approach and success stories, resonating with individuals globally and drawing them toward holistic nutrition guidance that felt personal and genuine.

Streamlining Success: Operational Efficiency: Embracing technology, Ava streamlined operations with advanced CRM and scheduling tools, ensuring each client felt seen and valued. Automation supported growth but never at the expense of the personal touch that was Ava's signature.

Virtual Gatherings: Strengthening Bonds: Ava hosted virtual wellness retreats, bringing together holistic health experts and her growing community. These events were more than educational—they were a celebration of collective well-being, strengthening the bonds within her community.

Giving Back: Philanthropy as Growth: Ava launched a wellness grant program to support those with limited access to holistic health resources. This initiative amplified her social impact, reinforcing her commitment to accessible wellness for all.

Leading with Innovation: Staying Ahead: Dedicated to continuous learning, Ava stayed at the forefront of wellness trends, ensuring "Nourish & Flourish" remained an authoritative voice in holistic health. Innovation was her compass, guiding the expansion of her offerings and the evolution of her practice.

Ava's journey to scaling "Nourish & Flourish" to seven figures was a testament to the power of dreaming big while staying grounded in authenticity. Each strategic addition, from digital courses to community-building efforts, was infused with her original mission: to heal and inspire. As her practice grew, so did her impact, reaching far beyond financial metrics to touch lives globally. Ava proved that with vision, dedication, and a heart centered on wellness, scaling to seven figures while maintaining the soul of your practice is not just possible—it's transformative.

Chapter 8 Intentions and Reflective Questions

Marketing with Authenticity: Effective Branding and Marketing Strategies That Resonate with Your Core Audience

Intent:

To inspire holistic health professionals to craft and implement marketing and branding strategies that are genuine, transparent, and reflective of their core values, thereby establishing deep connections with their target audience and fostering a loyal client base.

- What are the core values and messages of my holistic practice that differentiate it in the wellness market?
- How can I weave these core messages into every aspect of my marketing to ensure consistency and authenticity?

Understanding Your Audience:

- Who is my ideal client, and what specific needs, preferences, and values do they have that my practice addresses?
- How can I better understand and connect with my audience on a personal level through my marketing efforts?

Choosing the Right Marketing Channels:

- Which marketing channels (social media, email, blogs, etc.) are most effective in reaching my target audience, and why?
- How can I utilize these channels in a way that feels authentic and engages my audience meaningfully?

Creating Engaging Content:

- What types of content (educational, inspirational, case studies, testimonials) can I create that will resonate with my audience and provide real value?
- How can I ensure my content reflects the holistic principles and authenticity of my practice?

Leveraging Client Testimonials and Stories:

- How can I encourage my satisfied clients to share their stories and experiences in a way that feels genuine and respects their privacy?
- What strategies can I use to showcase these testimonials to help potential clients understand the impact of my work?

Building Community Around Your Brand:

- What initiatives can I undertake to foster a sense of community among my clients and within the broader wellness sphere?
- How can community-building activities enhance my practice's visibility and credibility?

Measuring Marketing Effectiveness:

- What metrics and feedback mechanisms can I use to gauge the effectiveness of my marketing strategies?
- How can I adapt and refine my marketing approach based on this feedback to ensure it remains authentic and resonates with my audience?

Ethical Marketing Practices:

- How can I ensure my marketing practices uphold the highest ethical standards, particularly regarding claims about the benefits of my services?
- What steps can I take to maintain transparency and honesty in all my marketing and advertising efforts?

Reflecting on these questions encourages holistic health professionals to approach marketing not just as a means to attract clients but as an opportunity to genuinely connect with individuals seeking guidance and support in their wellness journeys. By prioritizing authenticity in your branding and marketing strategies, you can create lasting relationships with your audience, built on trust and shared values, thereby establishing a strong, reputable presence in the holistic health community.

PART - 4

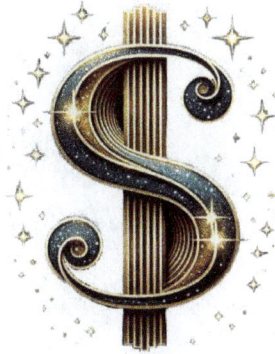

Enhancing Personal and Community Well-being

Chapter 9

Self-Care for the Holistic Entrepreneur: Prioritizing Your Wellness as the Foundation of Your Business's Success

As holistic practitioners, you dedicate yourselves to nurturing the well-being of others. Yet, it's crucial to remember that your ability to heal and inspire is deeply connected to your own state of wellness. Whether you're just embarking on your holistic journey or are an established practitioner, integrating self-care into your routine is not just beneficial—it's essential for the sustainability and growth of your business. This chapter explores the significance of self-care for holistic entrepreneurs and offers practical strategies to incorporate it into your life.

1. Understanding the Role of Self-Care

Self-care is the foundation upon which the success of your practice is built. It enhances your physical, mental, and emotional resilience, enabling you to serve your clients with energy, compassion, and creativity. Ignoring self-care can lead to burnout, diminishing your capacity to make a positive impact.

2. Physical Well-being

- Regular Movement: Incorporate physical activity into your daily routine, whether it's yoga, walking, or any exercise that you enjoy. Physical well-being directly influences energy levels and overall health.
- Nourishing Diet: Practice what you preach by choosing nutritious foods that fuel your body and mind. A balanced diet supports cognitive function and emotional stability.
- Adequate Rest: Prioritize sleep and rest. Quality sleep is crucial for recovery, decision-making, and maintaining emotional balance.

3. Mental and Emotional Well-being

- Mindfulness Practices: Engage in mindfulness practices such as meditation, deep breathing, or journaling. These practices can help manage stress, enhance focus, and foster a sense of inner peace.
- Setting Boundaries: Learn to set healthy boundaries between work and personal life. It's essential to have time to recharge and engage in activities that bring you joy outside of work.

4. Building a Supportive Community

- Seek Support: Cultivate a network of peers, mentors, or a mastermind group. Sharing experiences and seeking advice can provide emotional support and inspire new ideas.
- Give Back: Volunteering or offering community workshops can be fulfilling and reinforce your connection to your mission, reminding you of the "why" behind your work.

5. Regular Self-Reflection

- Check-in with Yourself: Regularly assess your physical, mental, and emotional states. Being aware of your needs allows you to address them proactively.
- Celebrate Achievements: Acknowledge your successes, no matter how small. Celebrating achievements fosters a positive mindset and motivates continued effort.

6. Integrating Self-Care into Business Planning

- Schedule Self-Care: Treat self-care as non-negotiable appointments in your calendar. By scheduling these activities, you ensure they are a priority.
- Delegate and Outsource: Recognize when to delegate tasks or outsource work to maintain your well-being. This can free up time for self-care and strategic business activities.

For holistic entrepreneurs, self-care is not a luxury—it's a critical component of professional practice. By prioritizing your wellness, you not only safeguard your health but also ensure the vitality and longevity of your business. Remember, the most profound impact you can have on your clients starts with the care you give yourself. As you grow your practice, let self-care be the light that guides your journey, illuminating the path to success for both you and your community.

Chapter 9 Intentions and Reflective Questions

Self-Care for the Holistic Entrepreneur: Prioritizing Your Wellness as the Foundation of Your Business's Success

Intent:

To emphasize the importance of self-care for holistic entrepreneurs, highlighting how their personal well-being directly impacts the success and vibrancy of their business, and providing strategies to integrate self-care into their daily routines.

Reflective Questions: *Recognizing the Role of Self-Care*

- How does my current level of self-care affect my energy, creativity, and ability to lead my holistic practice?
- In what ways can improving my self-care practices enhance the overall success and health of my business?

Identifying Personal Self-Care Needs:

- What specific aspects of my physical, mental, and emotional well-being am I currently neglecting?
- How can I create a personalized self-care plan that addresses these needs while fitting into my busy schedule as an entrepreneur?

Creating a Self-Care Routine:

- What daily or weekly self-care practices can I commit to that will support my well-being and business goals?
- How can I ensure that my self-care routine is flexible enough to adapt to changing needs and circumstances?

Setting Boundaries for Work-Life Balance:

- What boundaries do I need to establish to protect my time for self-care and prevent burnout?
- How can I communicate these boundaries effectively to clients, employees, and colleagues to ensure they are respected?

Leveraging Resources for Self-Care:

- What resources (apps, books, courses, communities) are available to support my self-care journey as a holistic entrepreneur?
- How can I incorporate these resources into my self-care strategy without feeling overwhelmed or overcommitted?

Self-Care as a Model for Clients:

- How does my commitment to self-care serve as a model for my clients and reinforce the holistic principles of my practice?

- In what ways can I share my self-care journey to inspire and encourage my clients to prioritize their well-being?

Overcoming Obstacles to Self-Care:

- What are the biggest challenges I face in maintaining a consistent self-care practice, and how can I address them?
- How can I remain motivated to prioritize self-care even when faced with pressing business demands or personal setbacks?

Evaluating and Adjusting Your Self-Care Plan:

- How will I assess the effectiveness of my self-care plan in improving my well-being and business success?
- What criteria will I use to decide when it's time to adjust my self-care practices to better meet my needs?

Reflecting on these questions enables holistic entrepreneurs to recognize self-care as an indispensable part of their business strategy. By committing to their personal well-being, they not only enhance their capacity to serve others but also set a powerful example of holistic living for their clients, employees, and the broader community. Prioritizing self-care is not a luxury—it's a necessity for sustaining a successful, fulfilling holistic practice.

Chapter 10

Cultivating Community and Collaboration: Building Networks and Fostering Relationships for Mutual Growth

In the realm of holistic wellness, the strength of your practice often lies in the community you build around it and the collaborations you foster. Whether you're at the beginning of your holistic journey or are seeking to enhance your established practice, nurturing a network of like-minded individuals and professionals can catalyze your growth and extend your impact. This chapter delves into strategies for cultivating a thriving community and meaningful collaborations that support mutual growth.

1. The Power of Community

A strong community not only supports your business but also amplifies the principles of holistic wellness by fostering a sense of belonging and collective well-being. Engaging with your community—be it clients, fellow practitioners, or broader wellness enthusiasts—creates a supportive ecosystem where everyone contributes to and benefits from shared knowledge, experiences, and resources.

2. Engaging Your Client Community

- Create Interactive Platforms: Utilize social media, forums, or your website to create spaces where your clients can interact, share their stories, and support each other. This interaction fosters a sense of belonging and loyalty to your brand.
- Host Events: Organize workshops, seminars, or retreats that bring your clients together. These events are not just educational; they're opportunities for individuals to connect, forming a community centered around your practice.

3. Fostering Professional Collaborations

- Network with Peers: Attend conferences, join professional associations, or participate in online groups related to holistic health. These networks can be invaluable sources of support, advice, and referrals.

- Collaborate on Projects: Identify practitioners or businesses whose offerings complement yours. Joint ventures, whether they're co-hosted events or collaborative service packages, can broaden your reach and offer your clients a more comprehensive wellness experience.

4. Building Partnerships Beyond the Wellness Industry

- Explore Cross-Industry Opportunities: Look for partnership opportunities with businesses outside the traditional wellness sphere but with aligned values. This could include local organic farms, eco-friendly product companies, or corporate wellness programs. Such partnerships can introduce your practice to new audiences and add value to your offerings.

5. Leveraging Technology to Build Networks

- Utilize Digital Tools: Platforms like LinkedIn, Clubhouse, or specialized wellness apps can help you connect with other professionals and potential clients worldwide. Sharing insights, participating in discussions, and showcasing your expertise can attract collaborations and grow your community.

6. Contributing to the Greater Good

- Initiate or Join Collective Efforts: Engage in or support initiatives that aim to improve community health, environmental sustainability, or social well-being. These efforts not only contribute to your mission but also position your practice as a force for positive change.

7. Nurturing Relationships

- Maintain Regular Communication: Keep in touch with your network through newsletters, personal messages, or social media updates. Regular communication keeps relationships warm and opens the door for future collaborations.

- Offer Value: Always look for ways to provide value to your network, whether through sharing resources, offering advice, or giving referrals. The more you give, the more you'll receive in return.

Cultivating a strong community and fostering collaborations are foundational to scaling your holistic wellness practice. By building networks and nurturing relationships, you not only enhance your own growth but also contribute to the broader ecosystem of wellness. Remember, the path to success in holistic health is one best walked with others, where collaboration, support, and shared visions pave the way for mutual growth and transformative impact.

Chapter 10

Intentions and

Reflective Questions

Cultivating Community and Collaboration: Building Networks and Fostering Relationships for Mutual Growth

Intent:

To inspire holistic entrepreneurs to actively engage in community building and collaboration, recognizing the power of networks and relationships in amplifying their impact, driving growth, and fostering a supportive ecosystem for mutual success.

Reflective Questions: *Assessing Community Engagement*

- How connected do I currently feel to the holistic health community and my professional network?
- What steps can I take to deepen my engagement and presence within these communities?

Identifying Potential Collaborative Opportunities:

- What opportunities exist for collaboration within my network that could benefit my practice and others involved?
- How can I initiate collaborations that are aligned with my values and the needs of my community?

Building Meaningful Relationships:

- What strategies can I implement to build more meaningful and supportive relationships within my professional network?
- How can I ensure that these relationships are mutually beneficial and based on a genuine desire for mutual growth?

Leveraging Social Media and Online Platforms:

- How effectively am I using social media and online platforms to connect with peers, mentors, and potential collaborators?
- What content or initiatives could I share online to foster a sense of community and open doors to new collaborations?

Participating in Community Events:

- What role can I play in local and online community events, workshops, or conferences to enhance my network and visibility?
- How can participating in or hosting these events contribute to the growth of my practice and the holistic health community?

Creating a Culture of Collaboration:

- How can I foster a culture of collaboration and openness within my practice and among my professional contacts?

- What are the benefits of prioritizing collaboration over competition in the holistic health field?

Navigating Challenges in Collaboration:

- What potential challenges might I face in seeking out or maintaining collaborative relationships, and how can I address them?
- How can I ensure that collaborations remain aligned with my practice's mission and the collective goals of those involved?

Measuring the Impact of Community and Collaboration:

- How will I assess the impact of my community engagement and collaborative efforts on my practice and personal growth?
- What indicators will show me that these efforts are contributing to a stronger, more supportive holistic health ecosystem?

Reflecting on these questions encourages holistic entrepreneurs to view community building and collaboration not as optional extras but as essential components of a successful practice. By investing in networks and relationships, you not only enhance your own practice's growth and resilience but also contribute to the collective strength and vitality of the holistic health community, creating a ripple effect of wellness and support that extends far beyond your own endeavors.

PART -5

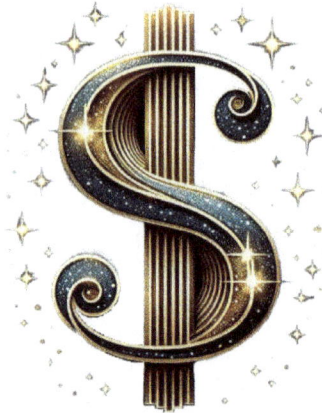

Advanced

Practices and

Innovation

Chapter 11

Leveraging Technology in Wellness: Incorporating Digital Tools and Platforms to Enhance Your Business and Practice

In today's rapidly evolving digital landscape, technology offers unprecedented opportunities to expand and enrich holistic wellness practices. From new practitioners to seasoned experts aiming to scale their businesses, leveraging technology can streamline operations, broaden reach, and provide innovative solutions to clients. This chapter explores how integrating digital tools and platforms can transform your holistic wellness practice, driving growth and fostering a deeper connection with your community.

1. Digital Presence and Branding

- Optimized Website: Your website is often the first point of contact with potential clients. Ensure it reflects your brand's essence, is easy to navigate, and is optimized for search engines to increase visibility.
- Social Media: Utilize social media platforms to share valuable content, engage with your audience, and showcase your expertise. Platforms like Instagram, Facebook, and YouTube are powerful tools for building community and driving awareness.

2. Virtual Consultations and Services

- Telehealth Platforms: Offer virtual consultations and services through secure telehealth platforms. This not only extends your reach to clients who are geographically distant but also adds a layer of convenience for those seeking flexible wellness solutions.

3. Online Courses and Workshops

- E-Learning Platforms: Develop and host online courses or workshops on topics related to your expertise. Digital learning platforms can help you reach a global audience, providing scalable passive income streams while educating and empowering clients.

4. Mobile Wellness Apps

- App Development: Consider developing a mobile app that complements your services. Whether it's for booking appointments, providing personalized wellness plans, or offering guided meditation sessions, a mobile app can enhance client engagement and support.

5. Automation and Efficiency

- Automated Booking and Scheduling: Implement online booking and scheduling tools to streamline appointment management. Automation saves time for both you and your clients, improving the overall experience.

- Client Management Systems: Use CRM (Customer Relationship Management) systems to manage client information, communication, and progress tracking. A robust CRM system can help personalize client interactions and improve retention.

6. Wearable Technology and Health Tracking

- Integration with Wearables: Collaborate with wearable technology that tracks physical activity, sleep patterns, or stress levels. Integrating this data can provide insights into your clients' wellness journeys, allowing for more personalized recommendations.

7. Virtual Reality and Wellness Experiences

- Innovative Wellness Experiences: Explore the use of virtual reality (VR) to create immersive wellness experiences, such as guided meditations or virtual nature walks. VR offers novel ways to support relaxation and stress relief.

8. Staying Ahead with Continuous Learning

- Digital Literacy: Keep abreast of technological advancements and digital marketing trends. Continuous learning ensures your practice remains relevant and competitive in the digital age.

9. Ethical Considerations and Data Security

- Privacy and Security: With the incorporation of digital tools, ensuring the privacy and security of client data is paramount. Adhere to best practices and legal requirements to protect sensitive information.

Integrating technology into your holistic wellness practice isn't just about keeping up with trends—it's about actively seeking ways to enhance the value you provide to your clients. From expanding your reach through digital platforms to enriching client experiences with innovative tools, technology offers a myriad of opportunities to grow your practice and deepen your impact. As you explore these digital avenues, remember to balance innovation with the personal touch and authenticity that lie at the heart of holistic wellness.

Chapter 11
Intentions and
Reflective Questions

Leveraging Technology in Wellness: Incorporating Digital Tools and Platforms to Enhance Your Business and Practice

Intent:

To guide holistic health professionals in effectively utilizing digital tools and platforms, aiming to optimize their business operations, expand their reach, and enrich the client experience, all while maintaining the integrity of their holistic practice.

Reflective Questions: *Evaluating Digital Needs*

- Which aspects of my practice could benefit most from digital enhancement or automation?
- How can I ensure that the digital tools I choose align with my holistic principles and the personal touch I value in my practice?

Exploring Digital Tools:

- What are the current leading digital tools and platforms in wellness, and how could they be applied within my practice?
- How can I stay informed about new technological advancements relevant to the holistic health field?

Enhancing Client Experience:

- In what ways can technology improve the experience for my clients, from initial contact through to ongoing support?
- How can I use technology to foster a sense of community and connection among my clients, even in a digital space?

Streamlining Operations:

- Which operational processes in my practice could be streamlined or improved through technology, such as booking systems, client management, or payment processing?
- What steps can I take to ensure the security and privacy of client data when using these digital tools?

Digital Marketing Strategies:

- How can I leverage digital marketing tools to effectively communicate my holistic health message and reach a wider audience?
- What are the most effective ways to measure the success of my digital marketing efforts and adjust strategies accordingly?

Creating Online Content:

- What types of online content (blogs, videos, online courses) can I create that will provide value to my audience and draw interest to my practice?

- How can I ensure that my online content remains authentic and reflective of my holistic approach?

Telehealth and Remote Services:

- How can I incorporate telehealth services into my practice in a way that complements my in-person offerings?
- What considerations should I keep in mind to maintain the effectiveness and personal connection of my services when delivered remotely?

Overcoming Technological Challenges:

- What are the most common technological challenges I might face, and how can I prepare for or address them?
- How can I seek out support or resources to navigate the digital aspects of running a holistic health practice effectively?

Reflecting on these questions helps holistic health professionals thoughtfully integrate technology into their practice, enhancing efficiency, reach, and client satisfaction without compromising the essence of their holistic approach. By strategically leveraging digital tools and platforms, you can not only streamline your operations but also create new pathways to connect with and support your clients in their wellness journeys.

Chapter 12

Innovative Wellness Trends: Staying Ahead with the Latest in Holistic Health and Wellness

The field of holistic health and wellness is continually evolving, driven by new research, emerging practices, and technological advancements. Staying informed about the latest trends is essential for both new and experienced practitioners aiming to provide the most effective and innovative care to their clients. This chapter delves into the importance of keeping pace with wellness trends and offers guidance on integrating these innovations into your practice for enhanced growth and client satisfaction.

1. Personalized Wellness Plans

- Precision Nutrition and Genomics: Tailoring wellness and nutritional advice based on genetic information can provide personalized health strategies for clients, offering targeted solutions for their unique needs.
- Wearable Health Technology: The data collected from wearable devices can inform personalized wellness plans, tracking everything from sleep patterns to physical activity, and offering insights into holistic health management.

2. Mental Health and Mindfulness

- Digital Mindfulness Solutions: With a growing emphasis on mental health, integrating digital mindfulness and meditation apps into your offerings can support clients' mental well-being alongside physical health.
- Psycho-Spiritual Practices: Techniques that blend psychological and spiritual approaches, such as breathwork and guided visualization, are gaining traction for their effectiveness in promoting mental and emotional balance.

3. Eco-wellness and Sustainability

- Green Spaces and Biophilic Design: Incorporating nature into wellness practices and spaces can enhance mental well-being and stress reduction. Practices are moving toward greener, more sustainable approaches that align with clients' values and environmental consciousness.
- Sustainable Wellness Products: Recommending or selling eco-friendly wellness products can reinforce your practice's commitment to sustainability and attract clients who value environmental stewardship.

4. Integrative and Functional Medicine

- Holistic Health Assessments: Combining conventional medical assessments with holistic evaluations to address the root causes of health issues, not just the symptoms, can offer comprehensive wellness solutions.
- Collaboration with Medical Professionals: Building networks with integrative and functional medicine practitioners can foster a collaborative approach to

client wellness, blending the best of conventional and holistic health practices.

5. Virtual Wellness Communities

- Online Support Groups: Leveraging social media and online platforms to create or join virtual wellness communities can provide additional support for clients, fostering a sense of belonging and shared purpose.
- Virtual Wellness Retreats: Hosting or participating in virtual wellness retreats can offer clients transformative experiences from the comfort of their homes, making wellness more accessible.

6. Continuing Education and Innovation

- Stay Informed: Regularly attend workshops, seminars, and conferences on holistic health to stay informed about the latest research and innovative practices.
- Experiment and Adapt: Don't be afraid to experiment with new techniques and technologies in your practice. Feedback from clients can guide the integration of these innovations for better health outcomes.

The landscape of holistic health and wellness is dynamic, with innovations that have the potential to deeply enrich your practice and enhance client well-being. By staying informed about and open to new trends, you position yourself as a forward-thinking practitioner capable of leading your clients through their wellness journeys with the most current and effective approaches. Remember, the integration of these trends should always align with the core values of holistic care—treating the whole person and fostering overall well-being.

Chapter 12
Intentions and
Reflective Questions

Innovative Wellness Trends: Staying Ahead with the Latest in Holistic Health and Wellness

Intent:

To equip holistic health professionals with the knowledge and tools to stay at the forefront of emerging wellness trends, enabling them to innovate within their practices, meet evolving client needs, and maintain a competitive edge in the holistic health industry.

Reflective Questions: *Identifying Trends*

- How can I regularly research and identify emerging trends in holistic health and wellness that are relevant to my practice?
- What are the most reliable sources of information for staying updated on these trends?

Evaluating Relevance and Alignment:

- How can I critically assess new wellness trends to determine their relevance to my practice and alignment with my holistic values?
- What criteria should I use to decide whether to integrate a new trend into my services or offerings?

Adapting to Client Needs:

- How can understanding current wellness trends help me better address the changing needs and interests of my clients?
- In what ways can I involve my clients in the process of exploring and implementing new wellness practices?

Innovation and Experimentation:

- What strategies can I employ to foster a culture of innovation and experimentation within my practice?
- How can I balance the excitement of trying new trends with the need to ensure they are safe, effective, and evidence-based?

Collaborating on Trend Integration:

- How can collaboration with other holistic health professionals or experts in specific wellness trends enhance my ability to integrate these trends into my practice effectively?
- What partnerships or networks could support my growth and learning in this area?

Marketing New Trends:

- How can I effectively communicate and market newly integrated wellness trends to my existing and potential clients?
- What messaging strategies can ensure that the introduction of new trends is seen as an enhancement

to my holistic approach rather than a departure from it?

Measuring Impact and Success:

- What metrics or feedback mechanisms can I use to evaluate the impact of integrating new wellness trends into my practice?
- How will I determine the success of these innovations in terms of client satisfaction, outcomes, and business growth?

Continual Learning and Growth:

- How can I commit to ongoing learning and professional development to stay ahead in the rapidly evolving field of holistic health?
- What habits or practices can I cultivate to ensure that my approach remains fresh, informed, and innovative?

Reflecting on these questions encourages holistic health professionals to actively engage with the latest trends in wellness, viewing them as opportunities for growth, differentiation, and enhanced client service. By staying informed, critically assessing relevance, and thoughtfully integrating new practices, you can ensure that your holistic health practice remains dynamic, responsive, and at the cutting edge of wellness innovation.

PART-6

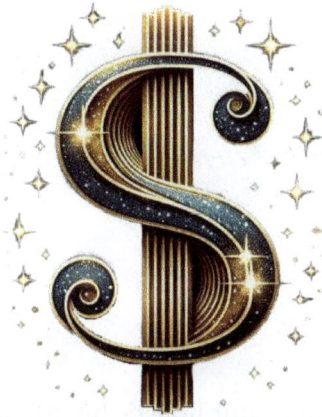

The Power of Intent in Action

Chapter 13

The Art of the Pitch: Mastering Pitch Presentations for Investors, with a Focus on Intent and Impact

As you consider scaling your holistic health business or seeking funding to bring your wellness vision to life, mastering the art of the pitch becomes essential. This chapter is designed to guide both new and seasoned practitioners through creating compelling pitch presentations that resonate with investors. The focus here is on blending intent—the core purpose and passion driving your business—with the tangible impact you aim to achieve, ensuring your pitch not only informs but also inspires.

1. Crafting Your Story

- Personal Journey: Begin with your journey into holistic health. Share your motivations, challenges, and the transformative moments that led you to where you are today. This narrative establishes a personal connection and highlights your commitment.

- Vision and Impact: Clearly articulate your vision for the future of your business and the broader impact you aim to make in the field of holistic health. This should reflect both your passion and the potential for positive change.

2. Demonstrating Market Need and Your Unique Solution

- Identify the Problem: Clearly define the specific problem or gap in the wellness market that your business addresses. This sets the stage for why your solution is necessary.

- Present Your Solution: Showcase how your holistic health practice offers a unique, effective solution. Highlight the innovative aspects of your approach and how it differs from existing offerings.

3. Showcasing Business Model and Strategy

- Revenue Streams: Detail how your business generates income, whether through services, products, or digital offerings. Be clear about pricing strategies, customer acquisition, and the scalability of your business model.

- Growth Strategy: Outline your plans for growth, including market expansion, new service development, or technological advancements. This demonstrates foresight and the potential for sustainable success.

4. Providing Evidence of Success and Impact

- Success Stories: Share testimonials or case studies that illustrate the positive outcomes your clients have experienced. This tangible evidence of impact can be compelling to investors.

- Metrics and Achievements: Include key performance indicators, such as client growth, retention rates, or revenue milestones, to quantify your business's success and potential.

5. Articulating the Ask

- Funding Needs: Be specific about the amount of funding you're seeking and how it will be used. Break down the allocation for product development, marketing, staffing, or other areas.
- Potential Returns: Discuss the potential returns on investment, both financially and in terms of social impact. Investors want to know what they stand to gain by supporting your venture.

6. Preparing for Q&A

- Anticipate Questions: Prepare answers to potential questions investors might have about your business, market strategies, or financial projections. This preparation shows thorough understanding and confidence.
- Feedback Loop: View questions as an opportunity to clarify and strengthen your pitch. Be open to feedback, as it can provide insights for refining your business approach.

Mastering the art of the pitch is about more than just selling your business idea; it's about sharing your passion for holistic health and the transformative impact you aim to make. By focusing on intent and impact, you can create a pitch that not only secures the investment you need but also champions the values at the heart of your practice. Remember, every pitch is a chance to bring others into your vision for a healthier, more holistic world.

Chapter 13

Intentions and Reflective Questions

The Art of the Pitch: Mastering Pitch Presentations for Investors, with a Focus on Intent and Impact

Intent:

To empower holistic health entrepreneurs with the skills and insights needed to craft compelling pitch presentations that effectively communicate the intent, impact, and investment potential of their businesses to potential investors.

Reflective Questions: *Clarifying Your Intent and Impact*

- How can I clearly articulate the core intent behind my holistic health business and the impact it aims to have on individuals and communities?
- In what ways can I demonstrate the alignment between my business's mission and the growing trends in wellness and sustainability that interest investors?

Understanding Investor Priorities:

- What are the key concerns and priorities of investors when evaluating health and wellness ventures?
- How can I tailor my pitch to address these priorities while staying true to my holistic principles?

Communicating Business Viability:

- How can I effectively present my business model, revenue streams, and growth strategy to showcase the financial viability and scalability of my venture?
- What evidence or data can I provide to support my claims and projections?

Storytelling and Emotional Connection:

- What storytelling techniques can I employ in my pitch to create an emotional connection with investors and make my business stand out?
- How can I share success stories or testimonials to illustrate the real-world impact of my services or products?

Preparing for Questions and Feedback:

- What are the most challenging questions I might face from investors, and how can I prepare thoughtful, confident responses?
- How can I remain open to feedback during the pitch process and use it constructively to refine my business proposition?

Visual and Presentation Skills:

- What visual aids or materials will enhance my pitch presentation and help convey my message more effectively?

- How can I improve my public speaking and presentation skills to engage investors fully and convey confidence in my business?

Building Relationships Beyond the Pitch:

- How can I use the pitch presentation as a starting point for building long-term relationships with investors, regardless of the immediate outcome?
- What steps can I take post-pitch to maintain communication and potentially explore future opportunities for collaboration?

Reflecting and Refining Post-Pitch:

- After delivering my pitch, how can I reflect on the experience to identify strengths and areas for improvement?
- What strategies can I implement to refine my pitch and business proposition based on the feedback and insights gained through the pitching process?

Reflecting on these questions prepares holistic health entrepreneurs to approach the pitching process as an opportunity to showcase their passion, professionalism, and the unique value of their ventures. Mastering the art of the pitch involves more than just presenting business facts; it's about weaving a compelling narrative that highlights your intent, impact, and the transformative potential of your holistic health business.

Chapter 14

Securing Investment for Holistic Ventures: Strategies for Attracting and Engaging with Investors Who Value Holistic Principles

In the evolving landscape of health and wellness, securing investment for holistic ventures requires a nuanced approach. It's about aligning your mission with investors who not only seek financial returns but also value the principles of holistic health. Whether you're pioneering a new wellness app or expanding a holistic therapy center, this chapter offers strategies to attract and engage with the right investors, ensuring your venture's growth is supported by partners who share your vision.

1. Identifying the Right Investors

- Research and Network: Start by researching investors known for supporting health and wellness ventures, especially those with a history of backing holistic or eco-conscious businesses. Utilize your professional network, attend industry events, and leverage online platforms to connect.
- Aligning Values: Look for investors who prioritize sustainability, wellness, and social impact alongside profitability. Their investment portfolio can offer clues about their alignment with your holistic principles.

2. Tailoring Your Pitch to Resonate

- Holistic Benefits: In your pitch, emphasize the holistic benefits of your venture. Highlight how your business contributes to physical, mental, and environmental well-being, providing a comprehensive view of its impact.
- Market Potential: Showcase the growing demand for holistic health solutions and sustainable practices. Use market data to illustrate the potential for significant returns on investment in the wellness sector.

3. Building a Compelling Narrative

- Your Story: Share your personal journey into holistic health and the founding story of your venture. Authentic stories can forge a deeper connection with investors who value purpose-driven businesses.
- Client Successes: Include testimonials or case studies that demonstrate the positive impact of your services or products on clients' well-being. Success stories can be powerful in illustrating the value and potential of your holistic venture.

4. Demonstrating Sustainability and Profitability

- Business Model: Clearly outline a business model that balances profitability with sustainability and holistic principles. Show how your venture can achieve financial success without compromising its core values.
- Growth Strategy: Present a clear, actionable growth strategy that highlights scalability and potential market expansion, reinforcing the long-term viability and attractiveness of your venture.

5. Leveraging Social Proof and Credentials

Endorsements: Gather endorsements from respected figures in the holistic health community or from satisfied clients. Social proof can enhance credibility and appeal to values-driven investors.

Certifications: Highlight any certifications or accreditations that underscore your commitment to quality, sustainability, or ethical business practices, adding to your venture's attractiveness.

6. Engaging with Transparency and Integrity

- Open Communication: Foster a culture of transparency in all interactions with potential investors. Open, honest communication builds trust and aligns expectations from the outset.
- Shared Vision: Focus on building relationships with investors who share your vision for a healthier, more holistic world. Mutual understanding and shared goals can lead to more fruitful partnerships.

Securing investment for holistic ventures is a journey of aligning your mission with investors who appreciate the value of holistic health and sustainability. By carefully selecting partners, tailoring your pitch, and demonstrating both the impact and profitability of your venture, you can attract investment that fuels growth while staying true to your principles. Remember, the right investors are those who believe in your vision and are committed to supporting the holistic well-being of individuals and the planet.

Chapter 14

Intentions and

Reflective Questions

Securing Investment for Holistic Ventures: Strategies for Attracting and Engaging with Investors Who Value Holistic Principles

Intent:

To guide holistic health entrepreneurs in identifying, attracting, and engaging with investors who not only provide financial backing but also share a commitment to holistic principles, ensuring a partnership that supports both business growth and the integrity of their holistic mission.

Reflective Questions: *Identifying Values-Aligned Investors*

- How can I identify investors who are genuinely interested in holistic health and wellness and whose values align with those of my venture?
- What networks, platforms, or communities can I tap into to connect with these potential investors?

Crafting a Values-Aligned Pitch:

- How can I ensure that my pitch effectively communicates the holistic principles at the core of my business, alongside its financial potential?
- In what ways can I highlight the alignment between my venture's mission and the personal or philanthropic interests of potential investors?

Demonstrating Impact and Viability:

- What specific examples of past success or impact can I present to demonstrate the effectiveness and viability of my holistic approach?
- How can I use data and research to support the growth potential and sustainability of my holistic venture?

Building Authentic Relationships:

- What strategies can I employ to build authentic and meaningful relationships with potential investors during the engagement process?
- How can I maintain transparency and open communication to foster trust and mutual respect?

Navigating Negotiations:

- How can I prepare for investment negotiations to ensure that the terms align with my holistic principles and business needs?
- What are my non-negotiables in an investment deal, and how can I effectively communicate these to potential investors?

Leveraging Social Proof:

- How can I leverage social proof, such as testimonials from clients or endorsements from well-respected figures in the holistic health community, to strengthen my case to investors?

- What other forms of social proof can I present to demonstrate the broader community support and demand for my holistic services or products?

Planning for Long-Term Partnership:

- Beyond the initial investment, what expectations do I have for my relationship with investors, and how can we collaborate for mutual benefit over the long term?
- How can I involve investors in the journey of my holistic venture in a way that keeps them engaged and supportive?

Learning from Rejections:

- How can I constructively handle rejections from potential investors, and what can I learn from these experiences to improve future engagements?
- What feedback mechanisms can I establish to gain insights from investors who decide not to invest in my venture?

Reflecting on these questions enables holistic health entrepreneurs to strategically approach the process of securing investment, focusing on partnerships that are not just financially beneficial but also deeply aligned with the holistic values and mission of their ventures. By cultivating relationships with investors who understand and support the principles of holistic health, entrepreneurs can ensure that their ventures grow in a way that stays true to their vision of promoting wellness and sustainability.

Chapter 15

Navigating Growth with Intent: Case Studies of Successful Holistic Entrepreneurs Who Have Scaled Their Businesses with Integrity

Scaling a holistic business requires more than just business acumen; it demands an unwavering commitment to integrity and the principles of holistic health. This chapter explores the journeys of several holistic entrepreneurs who have successfully scaled their ventures without compromising their core values. Through these case studies, you'll gain insights into the strategies, challenges, and triumphs that come with growing a holistic business with intent and integrity.

Case Study 1: The Holistic Wellness App

- Background: Maya, a seasoned meditation teacher, recognized the potential of digital platforms to expand her reach. She developed a wellness app that offered guided meditations, holistic health tips, and community features to support users' mental and physical health.

- Growth Strategy: Leveraging partnerships with wellness influencers and securing funding through investors who valued mental health initiatives, Maya expanded the app's features and user base. She maintained integrity by ensuring content was scientifically backed and culturally sensitive.

- Outcome: The app became a leading digital wellness platform, praised for its positive impact on users' well-being and its contribution to global mental health awareness.

Case Study 2: Sustainable Wellness Retreats

- Background: Carlos and Lina, passionate about environmental sustainability and holistic health, launched a series of wellness retreats that combined yoga, nutrition, and eco-education. They aimed to provide transformative experiences while fostering respect for the planet.

- Growth Strategy: By choosing eco-friendly venues and incorporating local community projects into retreat activities, they attracted attendees who shared their values. Strategic marketing and word-of-mouth recommendations fueled their growth.

- Outcome: Their retreats gained international acclaim for their authenticity, impactful experiences, and commitment to sustainability, leading to the expansion of their retreat locations and offerings.

Case Study 3: The Ethical Holistic Health Clinic

- Background: Dr. Nina, a naturopathic doctor, opened a clinic focused on integrative medicine, offering personalized holistic health plans. Her approach combined conventional medicine with alternative therapies, emphasizing the connection between body, mind, and environment.
- Growth Strategy: The clinic differentiated itself through rigorous practitioner training, a focus on research-backed treatments, and community health initiatives. Strategic partnerships with like-minded healthcare providers broadened their service offerings.
- Outcome: The clinic became a model for integrative medicine, respected for its ethical approach, comprehensive care, and contribution to advancing holistic health practices.

Case Study 4: Holistic Skincare Line

- Background: After years of research into natural remedies, Amina launched a holistic skincare line using ethically sourced, organic ingredients. Her products aimed to promote skin health without harmful chemicals, aligning with her beliefs in natural beauty and sustainability.

- Growth Strategy: Through transparent ingredient sourcing, environmentally friendly packaging, and educational marketing about skincare and health, Amina built a loyal customer base. Collaborations with eco-conscious influencers amplified her reach.

- Outcome: Amina's skincare line became a favorite among consumers seeking effective, ethical beauty solutions, leading to its expansion into international markets while maintaining its commitment to quality and sustainability.

These case studies of successful holistic entrepreneurs illuminate the path to scaling a business with integrity. They show that with a clear vision, a commitment to holistic principles, and strategic growth tactics, it's possible to expand your impact and achieve success without compromising the values at the heart of holistic health. Let these stories inspire you as you navigate the growth of your own holistic venture, reminding you that true success is measured not just in financial terms but in the positive change you bring to the world.

Chapter 15

Intentions and

Reflective Questions

Navigating Growth with Intent: Case Studies of Successful Holistic Entrepreneurs Who Have Scaled Their Businesses with Integrity

Intent:

To offer holistic health entrepreneurs inspiration and practical insights through real-world examples of successful holistic businesses that have managed to scale while maintaining their integrity and staying true to their core values and mission.

Reflective Questions: *Identifying with Success Stories*

- Which aspects of these case studies resonate most with my own journey and aspirations for my holistic venture?
- How do these success stories align with or challenge my perceptions of what it means to grow a holistic business with integrity?

Learning from Challenges and Solutions:

- What common challenges did these entrepreneurs face as they scaled their businesses, and how did they overcome them?
- How can I apply the lessons learned from their challenges and solutions to my own business growth strategy?

Maintaining Core Values During Growth:

- How did these entrepreneurs ensure that their core values and holistic principles remained at the forefront of their business operations as they scaled?

- What practices or policies can I implement in my own business to safeguard my core values during periods of growth?

Innovating While Staying True to Mission:

- In what ways did these case studies showcase innovation in product development, service delivery, or business model adaptation without straying from their holistic mission?
- How can I foster innovation within my own holistic venture while ensuring that new developments are consistent with my mission?

Engaging with the Community and Clients:

- How did these successful entrepreneurs use community engagement and client feedback to fuel their growth and enhance their services?
- What strategies can I use to deepen my engagement with my community and clients to support sustainable growth?

Building and Leading a Team with Intent:

- What approaches did these entrepreneurs take to build and lead teams that shared their vision and commitment to holistic principles?
- How can I attract, develop, and retain a team that will be instrumental in achieving my holistic business's growth objectives?

Reflecting on Financial and Ethical Growth:

- How did these case studies balance financial success with ethical considerations and social impact?
- What measures can I take to ensure that my business's growth not only benefits me financially but also contributes positively to societal well-being?

Continual Learning and Adaptation:

- What role did continual learning, mentorship, and adaptation play in the success of these holistic entrepreneurs?

- How can I cultivate a mindset of continual growth and openness to change as I navigate the expansion of my holistic venture?

Reflecting on these questions after reading the case studies provides a rich source of motivation and guidance for holistic health entrepreneurs embarking on or in the midst of scaling their businesses. These real-world examples highlight that growth, when approached with intent and adherence to holistic principles, can lead to substantial success without compromising the entrepreneur's mission or values. They underscore the importance of innovation, community, and ethical considerations in building a holistic venture that thrives.

Conclusion

Elevating Holistic and Alternative Medicine

As we reflect on the journey of holistic and alternative medicine, it's clear that the field stands at a pivotal moment. The stories shared, the strategies outlined, and the case studies of successful entrepreneurs within this text are more than just narratives and guidelines; they are beacons of inspiration, illuminating the path forward for holistic health practitioners at every stage of their entrepreneurial journey.

Reflecting on the Journey

The journey of holistic and alternative medicine is one marked by resilience, innovation, and a deep commitment to the well-being of individuals and the planet. It's a journey that has seen traditional practices gain recognition and acceptance within the broader health and wellness community, driven by a growing body of research and an increasing public demand for treatments that address the whole person—body, mind, and spirit.

As holistic practitioners and entrepreneurs, you've navigated challenges and seized opportunities, always with the intent to heal and transform lives. You've shown that it's possible to build successful, impactful businesses without losing sight of the core values that drew you to this field in the first place.

Envisioning the Future Impact

Looking to the future, the potential impact of holistic entrepreneurship is boundless. As society continues to grapple with the complexities of health and wellness in a rapidly changing world, the principles of holistic and alternative medicine—focusing on prevention, natural remedies, and the interconnectedness of all aspects of health—will play an increasingly vital role.

- Widening Acceptance and Integration: The integration of holistic practices into mainstream healthcare systems is poised to expand, offering patients a more comprehensive approach to health and well-being.

- Innovation and Technology: Advances in technology will continue to open new avenues for delivering holistic health solutions, from virtual wellness platforms to personalized health apps, making holistic care more accessible and effective.

- Global Wellness Movements: As awareness of environmental sustainability and mental health grows, holistic and alternative medicine will be at the forefront of global wellness movements, advocating for practices that nurture both individual and planetary health.

A Call to Action

As you stand at the forefront of this evolving field, remember that your work as holistic health practitioners and entrepreneurs is not just a profession—it's a calling. You have the power to shape the future of health and wellness, to bridge ancient wisdom with modern innovation, and to lead a global shift toward more holistic, sustainable ways of living.

Embrace this role with passion and purpose. Continue to learn, to innovate, and to collaborate. Most importantly, hold fast to the intent that drives you—the intent to heal, to empower, and to make a lasting impact on the world.

The journey ahead is filled with promise. Together, let's elevate holistic and alternative medicine to new heights, creating a healthier, more holistic future for all.

Conclusion

Intentions and

Reflective Questions

Setting Intentions for Your Journey Ahead

Intent:

To inspire readers to move beyond reflection into action, integrating the insights and strategies explored throughout the book into their holistic practices and personal growth plans. This section aims to galvanize holistic health entrepreneurs to take concrete steps toward scaling their businesses with integrity, purpose, and a commitment to wellness.

Reflective Questions: *Integration of Key Learnings*

- What are the top three insights or strategies from this book that resonated with me the most, and how can I begin integrating them into my holistic practice?
- How do these insights align with my current business challenges and opportunities for growth?

Personal and Professional Alignment:

- How has my understanding of my personal values and professional goals evolved after reading this book?
- In what ways can I ensure that my future business decisions and growth strategies continue to reflect this alignment?

Action Plan Development:

- Based on the strategies and case studies presented, what specific actions can I take in the next 3-6 months to move my holistic business toward greater success and impact?
- How will I measure the effectiveness of these actions, and what benchmarks will indicate progress?

Overcoming Potential Obstacles:

- What potential obstacles do I foresee in implementing the strategies discussed, and how can I proactively address them?
- Who in my network or community can support me in overcoming these challenges?

Continued Learning and Growth:

- How can I commit to ongoing learning and adaptation to stay ahead in the rapidly evolving field of holistic health and wellness entrepreneurship?
- What resources (books, courses, networks, mentors) can I explore to deepen my knowledge and skills?

Sharing and Collaboration:

- How can I share the insights and successes I achieve through applying this book's principles with my peers and broader community to foster collaboration and mutual growth?

- In what ways can I contribute to the holistic health community, reinforcing the cycle of learning, sharing, and growing together?

Reflection and Mindfulness:

- How will I incorporate regular reflection and mindfulness practices into my routine to ensure I remain grounded, focused, and aligned with my intent as I scale my business?
- What practices or rituals can help me stay connected to the core reason I embarked on this holistic entrepreneurial journey?

By contemplating these questions and setting clear intentions for the journey ahead, readers can close the book not just with a wealth of knowledge but with a concrete plan to apply that knowledge toward meaningful growth and impact. This final reflection encourages holistic health entrepreneurs to take inspired action, armed with the strategies, insights, and motivation to scale their practices beyond six figures while staying true to their mission of promoting wellness and holistic health.

Appendices

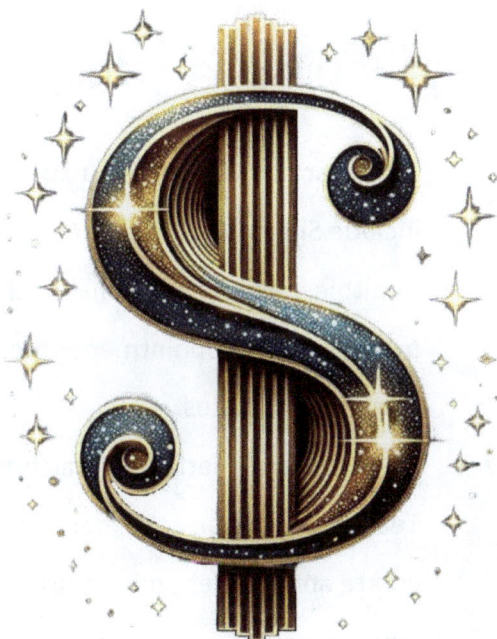

Appendix A: Resources and Tools for Holistic Entrepreneurs

This compilation includes a variety of resources to aid in the development, management, and growth of your holistic health business:

Digital Platforms and Software

- EHR/Practice Management Software: Examples include Simple Practice, Therapy Notes, and Healthie, offering solutions for client management, appointment scheduling, and telehealth services.
- Online Course Platforms: Platforms like Teachable, Kajabi, and Udemy can help you create and market online courses or workshops.
- Social Media Management Tools: Tools such as Hootsuite, Buffer, and Later assist in scheduling posts and managing your social media presence efficiently.

Business Development Resources

- Business Plan Templates: Templates from sources like the U.S. Small Business Administration (SBA) or SCORE can guide you in creating a comprehensive business plan.
- Marketing Guides: Resources from HubSpot Academy or the Digital Marketing Institute offer insights into digital marketing strategies tailored for health and wellness businesses.

Legal and Financial Tools

- Legal Document Templates: LegalZoom or Rocket Lawyer provide templates for essential legal documents, such as client consent forms and privacy policies.
- Financial Planning Tools: QuickBooks or FreshBooks offer accounting software tailored for small businesses, facilitating financial tracking and planning.

Books on Holistic Health Practices

- "The Complete Book of Ayurvedic Home Remedies" by Vasant Lad
    - A comprehensive guide to Ayurvedic remedies and holistic health practices.
- "Healing with Whole Foods: Asian Traditions and Modern Nutrition" by Paul Pitchford
    - Blends traditional Chinese medicine with modern nutritional science.
- "The Body Keeps the Score: Brain, Mind, and Body in the Healing of Trauma" by Bessel van der Kolk
    - Explores the impact of trauma on the body and mind, offering pathways to healing.

Books on Business Development

- "The E-Myth Revisited: Why Most Small Businesses Don't Work and What to Do About It" by Michael E. Gerber
    - Discusses common pitfalls in small business and offers insights for success.

- "Dare to Lead: Brave Work. Tough Conversations. Whole Hearts." by Brené Brown
  - Focuses on leadership that combines courage, compassion, and connection.
- "Building a StoryBrand: Clarify Your Message So Customers Will Listen" by Donald Miller
  - Guides businesses in clarifying their message and connecting with customers.

Journals

- "Journal of Holistic Nursing"
  - Offers research and insights into holistic nursing practices and patient care.
- "Global Advances in Health and Medicine"
  - Focuses on integrating traditional, complementary, and integrative health practices in patient care.
- "Journal of Alternative and Complementary Medicine"
  - Covers research, reviews, and perspectives on alternative and complementary medicine.

Websites

- National Center for Complementary and Integrative Health (NCCIH) nccih.nih.gov
    - Provides comprehensive information and research on complementary and integrative health practices.
- MindBodyGreen mindbodygreen.com
    - A lifestyle media brand dedicated to wellness tips, health news, and holistic practices.
- Holistic Entrepreneur Association holisticentrepreneurassociation.com
    - Offers resources, tools, and a community for holistic entrepreneurs looking to grow their businesses.

Appendix B: Glossary of Terms

This glossary defines key concepts and terms discussed throughout the guide, ensuring clarity and aiding in the deeper understanding of holistic health entrepreneurship:

- Holistic Health: An approach to well-being that considers the whole person—body, mind, and spirit—in the pursuit of optimal health and wellness.

- Integrative Medicine: A healing-oriented discipline that combines conventional medical treatments with alternative therapies to treat the whole person.

- Telehealth: The use of digital information and communication technologies, like computers and mobile devices, to access health care services remotely and manage your health care.

- EHR (Electronic Health Record): A digital version of a patient's paper chart, making information available instantly and securely to authorized users.

- CRM (Customer Relationship Management): A system for managing a company's interactions with current and potential clients, using data analysis to study large amounts of information.

- SEO (Search Engine Optimization): **The process of optimizing your online content so that a search engine likes to show it as a top result for searches of a certain keyword.**
- Sustainability: **Meeting the needs of the present without compromising the ability of future generations to meet their own needs, especially concerning environmental and social responsibility.**

By leveraging these resources and tools, and with a clear understanding of key terms, you're equipped to navigate the complexities of running and growing a holistic health business with confidence and integrity.

Bibliography

Holistic Health and Wellness

1. "The Encyclopedia of Natural Medicine" by Michael T. Murray and Joseph Pizzorno.
    a. A comprehensive guide on natural medicine and holistic treatments for a wide range of conditions.
2. "Healing Spaces: The Science of Place and Well-Being" by Esther M. Sternberg.
    a. Explores the impact of the physical environment on health and well-being.
3. "Integrative Nutrition: A Whole-Life Approach to Health and Happiness" by Joshua Rosenthal.
    a. Discusses the importance of nutrition and lifestyle choices in achieving overall health and wellness.

Business Development and Entrepreneurship

4. "The Lean Startup: How Today's Entrepreneurs Use Continuous Innovation to Create Radically Successful Businesses" by Eric Ries.
   - Offers a methodology for developing businesses and products through iterative design and customer feedback.
5. "Building a Story Brand: Clarify Your Message So Customers Will Listen" by Donald Miller.
   - Guides businesses in clarifying their message and connecting with customers through storytelling.
6. "Start with Why: How Great Leaders Inspire Everyone to Take Action" by Simon Sinek.
   - Explores the significance of understanding and communicating the 'why' behind your business.

Marketing and Digital Strategy

7. "Content Marketing for Nonprofits: A Communications Map for Engaging Your Community, Becoming a Favorite Cause, and Raising More Money" by Kivi Leroux Miller.

- Provides strategies for nonprofits and mission-driven businesses to effectively use content marketing.

8. "SEO 2021: Learn Search Engine Optimization with Smart Internet Marketing Strategies" by Adam Clarke.
   - A guide to current SEO strategies and practices for improving online visibility.

Legal and Ethical Considerations

9. "The Small Business Start-Up Kit: A Step-by-Step Legal Guide" by Peri Pakroo.
   - Offers legal and practical steps needed to start and run a successful small business.

10. "Ethics in Health Administration: A Practical Approach for Decision Makers" by Eileen E. Morrison.
    - Discusses ethical considerations and decision-making processes in health administration.

Sustainability and Environmental Health

11. "Sustainable Wellness: An Integrative Approach to Transform Your Mind, Body, and Spirit" by Matt Mumber and Heather Reed.

- Addresses wellness from a holistic and sustainable perspective, emphasizing the connection between personal health and environmental sustainability.

Mental Health and Mindfulness

12. "Wherever You Go, There You Are: Mindfulness Meditation in Everyday Life" by Jon Kabat-Zinn.
- Introduces the practice of mindfulness meditation and its application in daily life for stress reduction and emotional regulation.

Acknowledgments

In the creation of this comprehensive guide to holistic entrepreneurship, the journey from concept to completion has been enriched and made possible through the generous support, wisdom, and encouragement of numerous individuals and organizations. It is with deep gratitude that I extend my heartfelt thanks to all who have contributed to this endeavor.

First and foremost, my sincere appreciation goes to the myriad of holistic health practitioners and entrepreneurs whose stories and experiences form the backbone of this guide. Your willingness to share your journeys, challenges, and triumphs has provided invaluable insights and inspiration for others embarking on similar paths. Your dedication to healing and wellness illuminates every page.

A special thank you to the experts and mentors in the fields of holistic health, business development, and digital marketing who generously offered their time and expertise. Your guidance has been instrumental in shaping the content and ensuring the accuracy and relevance of the information presented.

I am also immensely grateful to the research and academic community, whose work continues to push the boundaries of our understanding of holistic health and entrepreneurship. The studies, papers, and texts cited in this guide reflect the depth of your contributions to the field.

To the editorial and design team, your talent and hard work have transformed a vision into a tangible resource. Your attention to detail, creativity, and commitment to excellence are evident on every page. Thank you for your patience, professionalism, and dedication to bringing this project to life.

My deepest appreciation extends to my family and friends for their unwavering support and encouragement throughout this process. Your belief in the importance of this work and your constant encouragement have been sources of strength and motivation.

Lastly, I extend my thanks to the holistic health community at large. Your passion for wellness, commitment to sustainable practices, and dedication to serving others continue to inspire and drive the evolution of holistic entrepreneurship. This guide is dedicated to you—all the practitioners, innovators, and dreamers who are making the world a healthier, more holistic place.

Thank you all for your invaluable contributions to this journey. Together, we are advancing the field of holistic health and entrepreneurship, paving the way for a future where wellness and business thrive in harmony.

Message from the Author

Dear Readers,

As I sit down to pen this message, my heart is full of gratitude and hope. The journey to compile this guide on holistic entrepreneurship has been as enriching as it has been enlightening. It's a reflection of not just my experiences but the collective wisdom and insights of a vibrant community dedicated to the noble cause of holistic health and wellness.

My path into the realm of holistic health was not a straight line; it was a journey marked by curiosity, learning, and a deep desire to understand the intricate connections between the mind, body, and spirit. Over the years, as I navigated the complexities of integrating holistic practices into a sustainable business model, I realized that my challenges were not unique.

Dr. Constance Santego 218

Many practitioners shared similar struggles—balancing the art of healing with the science of business, all while staying true to our core values.

This guide is born out of a desire to bridge that gap, to offer a roadmap that empowers holistic entrepreneurs to navigate their paths with confidence, integrity, and a sense of purpose. It is my hope that the strategies, case studies, and insights shared here will illuminate your journey, inspire innovation, and foster a deeper commitment to the transformative power of holistic health.

To all aspiring and established holistic entrepreneurs, this guide is for you. May it serve as a beacon, guiding you toward realizing your vision and making a meaningful impact in the world of health and wellness. Remember, the journey of holistic entrepreneurship is not just about building a successful business; it's about igniting change, fostering well-being, and contributing to a healthier, more holistic world.

As we look to the future, I am filled with optimism. The field of holistic health is evolving rapidly, and with it, the opportunities to make a profound difference in the lives of individuals and communities. Let us embrace these opportunities with open hearts and minds, committed to learning, growing, and innovating together.

Thank you for joining me on this journey. Your passion, dedication, and unwavering commitment to holistic health are what make this venture not just possible, but profoundly meaningful. Together, let's continue to elevate the practice of holistic and alternative medicine, transforming not only our own lives but those of the people we serve.

With deepest gratitude and warmest wishes,
Dr. Constance Santego

About the Author

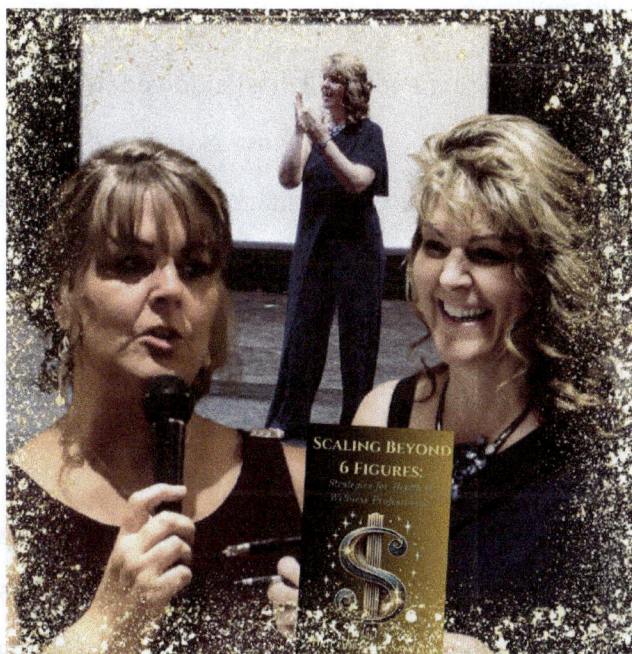

Dr. Constance Santego is not just a luminary in the fields of holistic health and entrepreneurship; she is a serial entrepreneur whose journey encompasses a broad spectrum of businesses, from industrial sewing and manufacturing to day spas, an accredited college, and even a café. This comprehensive guide to holistic entrepreneurship is infused with insights gleaned from her extensive experience in both traditional business realms and the wellness industry.

Her diverse entrepreneurial background, which includes running successful ventures in industrial sewing/manufacturing and retail, has endowed her with a unique perspective on business. These experiences have shaped her understanding of the market, consumer needs, and the importance of adaptability and innovation in business strategy. Dr. Santego's foray into the wellness sector, with her establishment of day spas and an accredited college focused on holistic health, further highlights her commitment to nurturing well-being in every aspect of life.

With a rich background that spans across natural medicine, spiritual guidance, and educational leadership, Dr. Santego has dedicated her life to fostering healing, growth, and transformation. Her holistic approach is deeply rooted in the belief that true wellness encompasses not only physical health but also the nourishment of the mind and spirit. This belief has been the cornerstone of her practice, teaching, and now, her latest literary contribution.

As an author, Dr. Santego invites readers into a world where the principles of holistic health meet the challenges and opportunities of entrepreneurship. Her writing is not just informative but a call to action, encouraging readers to embrace innovation, integrity, and intention in their ventures. Through her insights, she aims to light the path for aspiring and established holistic entrepreneurs, guiding them toward success that is both financially rewarding and spiritually fulfilling.

Beyond her written work, Dr. Santego is the founder of a holistic health and wellness school, a sanctuary for individuals seeking to deepen their understanding and practice of holistic living. Here, students are equipped not only with the knowledge to thrive in their personal health journeys but also with the skills to make a meaningful impact in the lives of others.

In her latest work, Dr. Santego has co-authored with ChatGPT to deliver a guide that is both a reflection of her expertise and a testament to her belief in the transformative power of holistic entrepreneurship. Her dedication to merging ancient wisdom with contemporary business practices shines through, offering a unique perspective that is both inspiring and pragmatic.

To explore more of Dr. Constance Santego's teachings, visit www.constancesantego.ca. Here, at the nexus of holistic health and entrepreneurial spirit, you will find a wealth of resources to support your journey toward creating a wellness business that is not only successful but also true to the values of holistic care.

Discover More

Embark on an Adventure with "Ikona – Discover Your Inner Genie"

Dive deeper into the world of empowerment and self-discovery with a range of offerings designed to inspire and transform. Explore the full spectrum of Constance Santego's motivational products, personalized coaching sessions, spiritual retreats, engaging live events, and enriching educational programs.

- Connect, Learn, and Grow:
- Website: Journey further into our resources and offerings at www.ConstanceSantego.ca.
- Instagram: Join our community @Constance_Santego for daily inspiration and insights.
- Facebook: Stay updated with the latest events and connect with like-minded individuals on Constance Santego's Facebook Page.

- YouTube: Subscribe to Constance Santego's YouTube Channel for free resources, meditations, and more to guide you on your path to self-improvement.

Your journey toward personal growth and enlightenment is just a click away. Discover the tools and support you need to unlock your potential and manifest your dreams.